Praise for *End Chronic Disease*

"The optimal approach for lifestyle-driven chronic disease is so vastly different than what we are used to in medicine, it takes a new breed of thinker and communicator to take us there. Kathleen is the perfect messenger for that mission."

— James Maskell, Founder of
Evolution of Medicine and Author
of *The Community Cure*

"Based on the principles of the individual's energetic state and their relationship to self, others, and the world around them, [Kathleen] invites the reader to engage in a simplified, but sound healing plan ladened with experiential wisdom. Clearly presented and scientifically backed, this simplified approach demonstrates how our microbiome-derived self is pivotal in achieving true health."

— Michelle Perro, MD, Pediatrician and Author
of What's *Making our Children Sick?*

END
CHRONIC
DISEASE

ALSO BY
KATHLEEN DICHIARA

The Hidden Connection:
Discover What's Keeping You
From Feeling Happy, Healthy
and Symptom-Free

END CHRONIC DISEASE

The Healing Power
of **Beliefs**, **Behaviors**,
and **Bacteria**

KATHLEEN DICHIARA

HAY HOUSE

HAY HOUSE, INC.
Carlsbad, California · New York City
London · Sydney · New Delhi

Published in the United States by: Hay House, Inc.: www.hay
house.com® • *Published in Australia by:* Hay House Australia
Pty. Ltd.: www.hayhouse.com.au • *Published in the United Kingdom by:* Hay House UK, Ltd.: www.hayhouse.co.uk • *Published
in India by:* Hay House Publishers India: www.hayhouse.co.in

Cover design: Howie Severson
Interior design: Julie Davison
Interior illustrations: Suzanne Darkan

**Cataloging-in-Publication Data is on file
at the Library of Congress.**

Tradepaper ISBN: 978-1-4019-5711-7
e-book ISBN: 978-1-4019-5712-4

10 9 8 7 6 5 4 3 2 1
1st edition, February 2020

Printed in the United States of America

This book is dedicated to my family and the ones brave enough to lead by example; thank you for modeling what's possible

CONTENTS

"If you trust in Nature, in what is simple in Nature, in the small Things that hardly anyone sees and that can so suddenly become huge, immeasurable; if you have this love for what is humble and try very simply, as someone who serves, to win the confidence of what seems poor: then everything will become easier for you, more coherent and somehow more reconciling, not in your conscious mind perhaps, which stays behind, astonished, but in your innermost awareness, awakeness, and knowledge."

— Rainer Maria Rilke, *Letters to a Young Poet*

INTRODUCTION

I had been firing on all cylinders for years, with a high-stress career in investor relations, a growing family, and recreational triathlon competitions on the side. But one day everything changed.

It was an early morning in August 2007. When I woke up and swung my legs to the side of the bed to head to the shower, I realized I couldn't bear any weight on my left leg. The days prior, I had been nursing a low-back pain—taking breaks to lie down in my office and asking my administrative assistant to run out for Advil, ice packs, and topical creams. But this was excruciating pain, and it was clear I wasn't going anywhere. What I didn't know then was that I would never return to that job that I loved. I had developed sudden-onset neuropathy caused by a compressed nerve in my lower back.

At the time, it was a mystery as to why this unexplained pain bubbled up to the surface, seemingly out of nowhere. This was particularly frustrating since I considered myself physically fit and there was no trauma or accident that set it off.

Despite my efforts, the pain got progressively worse. After six months of physical therapy and multiple rounds of steroid injections, I consulted with two surgeons. The first was an orthopedic surgeon who claimed to be an expert on the type of surgery I would require: an L4-L5 diskectomy and laminectomy. In this procedure a small portion of the bone in the spine is removed, and the disk in between the L4 and L5 vertebrae is released. This would relieve the pressure off the nerve and allow me to bear weight on my leg once again, something I was not able to do without pain. One thing the surgeon was very adamant about—the surgery would *not* remediate my low-back pain. This of course was a surprise to me, as this was the original symptom I had felt prior to nerve pain; but he insisted that back surgery provides no guarantee for back-pain relief. In fact, he said it was highly unlikely I would find relief as a result of the surgery.

The second doctor was a neurosurgeon. His diagnosis and prognosis seemed much grimmer. He recommended I also have a diskectomy/laminectomy in my lower back but included an additional diagnosis of degenerative disk disease, noting that my facet joints were deteriorating. The facet joints allow us to bend and twist, essentially keeping us flexible. I was only 35 years old—I certainly didn't expect this. His recommendation was to fuse together my lower vertebrae using metal rods, which I declined.

The entire process was overwhelming. I felt frustrated by the lack of options but also pressured to do something before I lost complete function of my left foot—which was starting to "drop" as a result of the compressed spinal nerve. At this point, I decided it was time to move ahead with surgery, choosing the more conservative orthopedic surgeon.

I specifically chose the first surgery slot of the day. I wanted my surgeon at his best—bright-eyed and ready to go. We had childcare lined up for the kids early that morning, and I was prepped and ready to be rolled in . . . except then I wasn't. We waited and waited. Finally, the anesthesiologist, who seemed to take a liking to my husband, Stephen, and me, noticed our frustration and told us they were having trouble getting the other surgery patient out of the operating room. When he saw the confused look on our faces, he explained that another surgery had been squeezed in before mine, only this was no ordinary patient. He was over 500 pounds. They needed special equipment to get him out of the operating room. I became visibly distraught. I began thinking of our kids and how the schedule delay would affect them. I started wondering how the stress of that complicated surgery would impact the staff and my surgeon. I contemplated leaving—but fearing that things would only get worse, I chose to proceed.

When I awoke, I knew something was terribly wrong; my legs wouldn't move. It was dark outside, and I was alone in the hospital room. I remember feeling stuck on my side, unable to turn over or reach for the buzzer to call for the nurse, so I reached for the room phone and dialed our home number. Stephen was home with the boys at this point—I told him to come back to the hospital immediately, which he did.

After running an MRI and ruling out a severed nerve in my spinal cord, the doctors eventually diagnosed me with Failed Back Surgery Syndrome, also known as "postprocedural complications following a laminectomy." This was my portal to a myriad of chronic diseases in the years to follow.

I was trapped inside a malfunctioning body. This led to the inevitable question, *Why me? How did this happen?* A common reaction when it feels as though your body has failed you.

What I didn't know then, but have since discovered, is that my body had not failed me. Instead, I had failed to properly manage the thousands of species of microbes that call my body home.

When disease and disability strike certain parts of the body, it's easy to feel like a victim and to focus on that *one* broken area of the body. But we are, in fact, super-organisms made up of trillions of microbes, the balance of which can have a significant impact on our overall health. Therefore, when one or more parts of the body stop working correctly, we have to take a look at the organism as a whole.

We are bacteria

The human body serves as a vessel for a collection of microbes. These microbes form an ecosystem that makes us who we are. This community of bacteria, fungi, viruses, and other microorganisms—form the *microbiome*. Microbes exist everywhere on and in the human body, although there are certain areas of the body that contain larger concentrations of microbes. The vast majority of them reside in the gastrointestinal tract, which harbors up to 1,000 different species.

So, what does the microbiome have to do with my poor response to surgery or ending chronic disease? Well, more than you think.

Until recently, this part of the hidden world within us was viewed primarily as a digestive tool that helped process our food and perhaps needed occasional fixing when digestive health went awry. When it came to fighting disease, we assigned the outcomes—good or bad—to our human genes. Surprisingly, we were wrong.

Our human genes only account for about 1 percent of our total genes, while our microbial genes make up the other 99 percent. While genes can predispose us to things like obesity, type 2 diabetes, or heart disease, *predisposed* is not the same as *predestined*. And how we live and behave is ultimately what regulates gene expression. In short, changing the types of microbes that live within us means we can change our genetic expression, which begins with how we choose to conduct our lives. The health of every organ and area of the human body relies on a healthy microbiome.

Healing is possible

Fortunately, it's not in my nature to give up. It was at this critical juncture in my life that I took a deep dive into nutrition, biology, physiology, and the rapidly evolving science of how food, lifestyle, and microbes affect our health, essentially making us who we are. Unsatisfied with the conventional medical approach, I embarked on a voracious study of the human body and its infinitesimally detailed choreography. It was three years postoperation, and I was already managing multiple chronic diseases—including fibromyalgia, chronic pain syndrome, irritable bowel syndrome (IBS), chronic myofascial syndrome, severe food allergies, and more.

I read hundreds of books, scoured the Internet, studied with experts, and used myself as a case study as I explored everything from the endocrine system to the digestive tract, vagus nerve pathways, and mitochondrial function. I learned how all the body's systems and our microbial organisms are designed to work in synergy, a cooperative army created to efficiently digest food and channel its energy and nutrients for optimal health. I'm not being dramatic when I say that what I learned saved my life.

During my recovery, I was also confronted with the declining health of the rest of my family. We now had three boys, and we were collectively managing 21 chronic diseases. As many families have experienced, it just happens. You're plugging along in life, dealing with each inflammatory dilemma—from skin rashes to food allergies—as it shows up. At the time one of our sons was on the autism spectrum, and I think, when you are raising a child on the spectrum, you become accustomed to multitasking co-morbid health conditions like digestive issues, sensory overload, and anxiety. But the more I learned about healing, the more I realized that these symptoms did not need to be permanent, nor did all the food allergies, eczema, and asthma my other boys were experiencing. Just because they were becoming common childhood conditions did not mean they were "normal."

On top of everything, my husband had suddenly developed gynecomastia. This excess development of breast tissue in males is often due to hormonal imbalances. It was all connected. We all needed to change. Did we change the quality of our food? You bet we did. But the changes that brought about lasting results happened in every area of our lives, in and outside of our home, and most importantly in our hearts and minds. You will find them on the pages of this book.

Today, I am a *walking* example of your ability to fully heal when you shift your mind-set, change your behaviors, and alter your microbiome for the better. We all healed, and so can you.

Our struggle served as the inspiration for my immersion into the field of functional nutrition, which focuses on finding the *root* cause of health imbalances. Through my clinical work as a nutrition practitioner and my own experience as a once chronically ill patient, I have been fascinated with the following question:

> *What differentiates those who overcome illness only to become stronger, more competent versions of themselves from those who stay in the vulnerable state of compromised health despite their best efforts?*

I felt compelled to write *End Chronic Disease* because my own healing journey was not a simple or straightforward path. As I searched for lasting solutions, I often found myself in a patient-practitioner loop that led to long-term disease "management." I worked with well-meaning practitioners whose compassionate care, though it did not cure my disease, was in many ways my lifeline during a very difficult time.

I eventually made enough progress and was able to wean myself away from strong pharmaceutical painkillers and other prescription drugs and therapies as I began seeking alternative approaches. However, I soon became overly dependent on disease-management care and the continued use of alternative remedies—rather than using remedies as a short-term bridge from the conventional medical approach of pharmaceuticals and surgery to a safer, more natural plan of supplements and therapies. My unsuccessful attempts to strip away the natural therapies or supplement regimens revealed that I was still very fragile, physically vulnerable, and, quite frankly, still sick. I was not as sick as I had once been, but I was clinging to a list of natural remedies to keep me alive and hold me together like glue. I was not thriving on my own.

It was becoming clear that, to truly condition the body to overcome illness, I would need to be less reactive and instead build resilience that would allow me to gain power and transform myself from my challenges.

Becoming flexible

These days, it's not uncommon to hear or read about resilience. That word is used frequently in the health and wellness space and in articles such as "25 Ways to Boost Resilience," in which psychologist Karen Horneffer-Ginter recommends things like taking an occasional walk in nature or a self-prescribed "time-out bath."

No doubt this is useful, timeless advice. I am certainly a huge advocate for self-care and time in nature (you'll hear more about that later). But is it adequate? How is it that such gentle, seemingly innocuous practices could possibly help us overcome chronic disease, fight depression or anxiety, or get us to a place where we can restore our overall wellness? On one hand, we are being reassured that positive thinking and affirmations are essential for healing. But on the other hand, most people are struggling with illnesses and conditions that can't necessarily be treated simply by looking "on the bright side."

Psychologists have also written about ways to boost resilience—especially when it comes to our emotional health—for decades, putting forth such insight as the following, from *Psychology Today* editor-at-large Hara Estroff Marano:

> *Resilient people do not let adversity define them. They find resilience by moving towards a goal beyond themselves, transcending pain and grief by perceiving bad times as a temporary state of affairs.*

A positive attitude is essential to a happy, healthy life; but I was seeking a different kind of resilience, outside of emotional fortitude and optimism. I wanted to know how we can cultivate *lasting* health that reconnects us to the ebbs and flows of the healing process, where we can still utilize advances in healthcare but *without* compromising the power and intelligence of nature. A version of wellness that honors the interconnectedness and natural rhythms of all ecosystems, including the ones inside of our bodies and outside of us in nature. One that acknowledges the importance of consistent, seemingly small behaviors as powerful agents of change. I suspected others were craving this too.

What I've learned is that those who master resilience tend to be conditioned for emotional and physical emergencies long before they ever strike. They are adept at accepting what comes at them with *flexibility* rather than rigidity. The old metaphor applies: resilient people are like bamboo in a hurricane—they bend rather than break. Or, if they do feel broken, there's still a part of them deep down that knows that they won't be broken forever and that things will get better. Their roots run deep, and they understand that broken branches can heal after the storm.

I believe that this flexibility is what's missing from our current approach to wellness. There is too much emphasis on quick fixes. We don't need another set of "rules" to live by. The field of health and wellness is full of them, and rarely do they lead to lasting, sustainable outcomes.

We don't need any more fixing. Instead, what we all need is to cultivate health through mastering the art and science of living in accordance with our body's true nature—one that honors our inner ecology. We have been led to believe that it is too hard to achieve optimal health and that the answers are too complex. They are not.

There truly is no mystery to good health. The real secret is your willingness to face whatever is holding you back. This book is an invitation to shift your perspective, your actions, and your ecology.

The healing cycle

For over a decade, I have been researching the impact of food and lifestyle on chronic disease—initially motivated by the pressing need to save my own life. Years later, as a nutrition practitioner, I would work with many clients seeking nutritional advice and counseling, but I could sense that their needs would never be satiated simply by changing their diet. They were asking for meal plans, supplements, and symptom relief for allergies, body aches, and more serious maladies, but what they were really describing was an intense disconnection to health—one that I recognized all too well, and that required *interconnected* healing.

Health is more than the absence of disease. I believe health is the capacity to adapt change so that we can maintain optimal physical, mental, and metabolic function throughout our life.

I discovered that our health is shaped by a cycle that follows this pattern: Our *beliefs* create our reality, and by extension, our beliefs drive our behavior. Our *behaviors*—for better or worse—become our lifestyle, which determines the quality and diversity of the microbes that call our body home. Collectively, these *bacteria* become our microbiome, which influences every aspect of our health, including our beliefs.

BELIEFS

BEHAVIORS

BACTERIA

Ending the pattern of chronic disease and becoming resilient is not about developing some kind of superhuman quality or biohacking your way to peak performance. It is simply a change in the way you approach your pursuit of health and well-being, a change that honors the adaptive, interconnected rhythm with which you were intended to live in sync with Mother Nature. And this approach is accessible to *everyone*, regardless of economic status. At the core, optimal health begins by adjusting the quality of your thoughts, the consistency of your daily habits, and the diversity of your inner and outer ecosystems.

This approach is for individuals who know that they are capable of healing but for some reason feel they have not yet "cracked the code." It's for those who have been pursuing transformation to reverse chronic diseases or conditions, or have been trying to optimize their health, and in doing so have read countless books, attended seminars, and gathered so much information that they are now citizen scientists—yet still have not reached their wellness goals. My hope is that this book will shatter the constraints that are holding you back from reaching your potential.

You can do it

At the core of optimal health is positive thinking—and I firmly believe that if you are reading this book, you have made the commitment to end chronic disease for yourself and the people you care about.

I also believe that in order for true healing and lasting change to occur, we need to tap into what connects us as individuals to our own bodies and our own minds, as well as to the health of the planet. It's a cyclical sequence, with each component linking to the next and each being of equal importance.

As we heal ourselves, we help to heal the people around us and the planet as a whole.

This book is intentionally pared down because I have come to learn that it is the simple things in life that are the most profound. With chronic diseases at an epidemic level and so many people suffering in the world, I want to reiterate that there is no magic bullet for the complex health problems that we face but that consistent, meaningful actions do make a big difference.

I also chose to lighten the *tone* of the book by incorporating illustrations because art invites us to open up in a different way than the written word does. I know for me, there is something about creativity that swings my heart wide open, a playfulness that invites me in. I chose Suzanne Darkan as the artist because we share a passion to serve humanity and improve the world—hers through artistic endeavors for mental health, and mine through nutritional education for those with chronic illness.

End Chronic Disease is structured in three parts: The first section, Beliefs, is designed to help you to let go of any limiting beliefs that may be holding you back from healing and shift your mind-set to pave a new path to wellness. The second section, Behaviors, offers sixteen practical habits designed to rebalance your lifestyle and build your inner ecology. And the third section, Bacteria, provides some of the key lessons from our microbial partners that will transform your understanding of the links between human health and our connection to nature and each other.

My intention is not for you to memorize or master the principles in this book but for you to consider the health of your whole body and incorporate this framework into your daily life to make way for optimal health.

Part I

BELIEFS

Your body cannot go where your mind is not willing to take you—how and what you think creates your reality. This means that your thoughts lay the groundwork for your lifestyle, and you can use your thoughts deliberately to improve your life and your health.

After overcoming my own health crisis, I found myself face-to-face with countless chronically sick individuals on their own personal quests to get well. I noticed a common thread: people believe that chronic diseases need to be medically "treated." Thus, they rely on interventions and medications to alleviate symptoms without tending to the underlying causes that produced those symptoms in the first place. This band-aid approach leads them down the path of using the same set of tools our health-care system uses to treat acute issues. Ultimately, they are left *managing* chronic disease instead of eliminating it.

The truth is, we have to create a different environment than the one that existed before the disease pattern occurred, and that starts with changing our mind-set.

Chronic disease is never singular. It is a sign that the body's ecology is breaking down (literally), which typically happens over a long period of time. By the time symptoms occur, we are already deep into the disease pattern. How chronic disease manifests for each of us is unique. Even the absence of a medical diagnosis does not necessarily equate to the presence of wellness. Many people do not develop chronic disease, but they are certainly not experiencing optimal health.

In order to use your thoughts and belief systems to heal, you need to first move the focus away from the confinements of your own problems, opening your awareness to the idea that your struggle with chronic disease is part of the larger dysfunctional global pattern that we all need to opt out of—for example, partaking in the highly processed food systems that are damaging to both our bodies and our planet is a surefire way to keep you sick.

This shift in your thinking will break you free from feeling isolated and defeated by your own illness. When you broaden your beliefs about what it means to truly cultivate long-term health, you can begin to see and feel your innate connection to the world—a world that is capable of change and goodness. And this sense of re-attachment fosters the beginning of the deep healing that we are all craving.

We live in a paradigm of seperation. The mind is often viewed seperatley from the body. A lot of people seek treatment to fix the body, while ignoring their mental and emotional quality of life. In Part I, we will explore the key areas where, in my interactions with individuals with chronic disease, limiting beliefs inevitably showed up at some stage in their illness. While the details of their self-talk were unique to their life experiences, the beliefs that repeatedly became the barriers to the healing process always fell into the same core buckets. I grouped my findings into six key areas: *values, wisdom, nourishment, intuition, emotions,* and *connection*. In each area, I have offered an alternative belief to serve as an anchor that I invite you to reconsider as a new framework to set the stage for optimizing health.

- Values: *Congruence creates harmony*
- Wisdom: *I am my own healer*
- Nourishment: *Food is information*
- Intuition: *Self-trust is my most powerful guide*
- Emotions: *Positive Feelings Recondition the Mind and Body to Heal*
- Connection: *The health of each is bound by the health of all*

Keep in mind, it is not my intention or goal in this book to define what your individual beliefs should be, for that is beyond what can be taught. Think of these beliefs as overarching themes to remove the blocks to your own awareness. They can be used as purposeful thoughts to prompt you to reconsider what it means for you to heal and/or live a healthy life. There is no way for me to define health for you without imposing my views on you. This would rob you of the ability to choose what matters to you and what wellness means in your own life. These beliefs are designed to allow you to explore your own life in a way that resets your unique path, particularly in the areas of your life that no longer serve you or are holding you back.

These should serve as "guardrails" for navigating a shift in mind-set, which will positively influence your lifestyle behaviors and ultimately regenerate your microbial ecology to foster resiliency. Keep in mind that the journey to cultivate health and end chronic disease has no set path, but I have found that each person has their own unique set of limiting beliefs about their capacity to heal that holds them back.

You must be willing to reprogram your thoughts and consider a different set of beliefs that will help you shift and strengthen your mind, body, and soul toward a life built for flexibility and the capacity for change. This is often referred to as the "mind-body approach," but I invite you to take it further and recognize that your thoughts and beliefs inform your health status.

Your journey to regenerating and sustaining long-term health starts here.

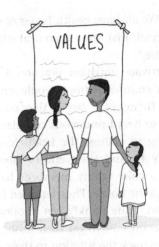

VALUES

Congruence Creates Harmony

The true foundation for regenerating health and achieving resilience is living in congruence. *Congruence* simply means that things make sense: there is an atmosphere of integrity and trust, which creates a safe haven in ourselves and in our environment. We all need to feel safe and secure to achieve optimal health.

People often ask me where to begin. Shortly after I finished giving a lecture on nutrition at the Soil & Nutrition Conference at Kripalu Center in the Berkshires of Massachusetts, a woman from the audience followed me out into the hallway and anxiously said, "My whole family is suffering. We all have health issues of some sort. But I have to fix myself first, then I can deal with everyone and everything else."

In my private nutrition practice, I had repeatedly heard similar comments from people who thought they had to "cure themselves" before they could help anyone else. I had also heard numerous complaints from mothers attempting to address the health concerns of their children only to find their efforts sabotaged by their husbands or a close family member's habit of bringing junk food into the house. They reported feeling defeated, exhausted, and, quite frankly, out of options. I would be asked for ideas on how to get their husbands "on board" or ways to fast-track the solution to their personal health crisis so they could muster the energy to somehow salvage the health of their children before the kids left for college.

Unfortunately, when you operate from the mind-set that your health, or the health of just one family member, must be mastered first or even alone, you are operating in a state of conflict. This can be confusing at a time when the self-care safety message reminds us, "In case of emergency, please put on your oxygen mask before helping others."

In our day-to-day lives, there is an interconnectedness between our own health as individuals and the health of our surrounding environment, which more specifically includes the people in it, especially family. It's nearly impossible for any individual to achieve optimal health—which arises from positive beliefs—when everyone around that person is operating with limiting beliefs and somewhat destructive behaviors.

In order for an individual in any household to achieve optimal health, it's critical for *everyone* in the household to get on board. Healing is a team sport. And you'll find you naturally pull each other up as you go along. Working together serves as a catalyst for transformation. "You're only as strong as your weakest link"—this idiom emphasizes that each individual's success, which in this case means health, is vital to the success of the entire group.

Congruence refers to "a state of agreeing," in which a person's values and beliefs are consistent with the way that individual lives his or her life. Congruence honors harmony and balance. A lack of congruence creates discord and internal tension. You achieve congruence when what goes on in your internal world is consistent with what you say and do in your external one. Your quality of life is a direct reflection of the standards you set for yourself and your family. When it comes to health, eating nourishing foods, exercising, meditating, spending time in nature, and getting proper sleep are obvious ways you can raise your standards for a better outcome. However, to support the health and healing of everyone in a household, you must establish positive values and goals that shift the vibration of the whole environment to that of harmony and alignment.

Here's another way to think of it: Companies develop mission statements, which, like values, help to guide them by defining *who they are* and *why they do what they do*. Values are usually fairly stable, yet they don't impose strict limits or rigid boundaries. As you move through life, your values will likely change. For example, your values may reflect different stages in your life: when getting married, faith or balance might be your focus, but that will change when it's time to grow your family. Staying in touch with your values is a lifelong commitment. You should continuously revisit your values, especially when you feel unbalanced or unstable and can't quite figure out why.

Ideally, your beliefs and values should be aligned with the way you carry out your daily activities and your vision for your life so that you are not operating in a constant state of conflict.

Chronic disease is an opportunity to unravel the truth about what is making us sick. In doing so, we begin to see the various contributors to disease and, more importantly, what defines health. When you begin to explore what matters to you—your values—you can create the life you want. This is how you use chronic disease as a *collective call to action.*

For example, you might find respite and healing near the ocean. You could make the powerful decision to discontinue the use of plastic water bottles and transition to stainless steel and glass products at home as a way to reduce your impact on the eight million metric tons of plastic that are thrown into the ocean every year. Plastic is bad for you and the planet.

Plastic water bottles contain hormone-disrupting toxins. Even if companies claim they nixed the bisphenol A (BPA), plastic is laced with other chemicals that seep into the water if bottles are exposed to heat or sit around for a long time. Studies show that bottled water—which often comes from the tap, not the peaceful mountain spring on the label—contains phthalates, mold, microbes, benzene, trihalomethanes, and even arsenic. And only recently did the FDA start regulating bottled water for *E. coli*. Inside the body, BPA acts like an estrogen—interfering with puberty in our developing boys and girls. It has also been linked to type 2 diabetes, obesity, and attention deficit hyperactivity disorder (ADHD). Even tiny amounts can trigger changes in the body that lead to serious health problems.

Exploring the role of environmental triggers and how these chemicals interfere with the bodies' function, especially metabolism and hormones, is one way to link your health goals to a greater vision for the world and make a powerful shift toward congruence. Imagine, the simple act to ditch disposable bottled water helps you live healthier and connects you to a movement for global sustainability. Plus, it's easy, and you'll save money.

Another area significantly impacted for anyone struggling to overcome chronic health challenges is *nutrition*. Many people abide by restrictive diets while their family members eat anything and everything. Oftentimes, family members who are free from the ravages of serious illness may not feel the need to change their diets simply because they feel they don't have to. Other times this is a choice to offset expenses associated with foods free from certain allergens or because the idea of making drastic changes for the entire family feels daunting.

But what if you shifted your beliefs about what it means to cultivate health and resilience for yourself and everyone around you? What if you saw this as an opportunity for the whole family to unite and grow, rather than a burden for one individual to overcome?

Sadly, more often than not, individuals who are ill are treated as "broken" and are expected to work through their health crises on their own, which often leads them to feelings of isolation, deprivation, suffering, and "being different" because they are sick. Because the values of the whole family unit have not shifted in alignment toward health, there is conflict. This is not an ideal healing environment—and it rarely brings about lasting change.

I have witnessed countless success stories in which families have made the bold choice to revisit their values and honor a more congruent path to supporting the health and healing of *everyone* in the family. With this approach the entire vibration shifts in alignment, and the outcomes are remarkable. This was certainly the experience in my family as well. Once we stopped addressing each individual ailment in isolation and realigned our lifestyle as a family, it was as if the goal of optimizing health of the whole family served as a stimulus for healing my oldest son and myself, as we were the most health-compromised at the time.

An important aspect of living in congruence is the understanding that you are living *your* truth, which will differ from the truths of other people you spend time with, such as friends and co-workers. Staying in alignment with your guiding principles will provide you with a sense of contentment and inner peace. When your behaviors and personal choices are aligned with your values, it creates a real sense of freedom and liberation about the way you live—both at home and out in the world—rather than resentment and frustration in social situations.

Congruence is being able to consistently say yes in life and knowing when to say no. It's also about being open to possibilities in life. The healing path comes with great challenges, and many people find that pursuing a healthy lifestyle in today's modern world is very difficult, at least socially.

You may discover, as I did, that adopting an organic, gluten-free diet all of the time makes you feel your best. However, if your dietary lifestyle becomes a wall to protect and isolate yourself, after some time you may find you feel you're in your own prison. Walls of self-preservation can also become the walls of self-confinement. Creating a safe haven should give a sense of confidence, not confinement, and provide a doorway to the world. It's a state of internal harmony that keeps you from feeling conflicted and confused about your lifestyle choices. An awesome feeling of inherent trust comes from people who are congruent. Whether you know it or not, congruence is often what attracts you to another person. People want to be around people who are in alignment. This does not mean we only choose people who share our same values and diets, but rather, we respect people who are living a life that is aligned with their own beliefs, even when their beliefs and values are different from ours.

Fortunately, you can cultivate congruence with practice. The first step is to clearly define your values and beliefs in areas of your life that are essential to you and your loved ones: your spirituality, your physical health, your career, your contribution to the world, your relationship to nature, and so on.

Congruence creates harmony: a coherence that sets the stage for true healing.

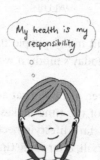

My health is my responsibility

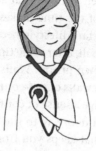

WISDOM

I Am My Own Healer

It is who you are and what you believe that heals you, not just what you learn, or what the doctors say, or the treatments you've been prescribed. Self-knowledge is a silence beneath all the words.

We're not limited to what we learned in high school or college—or even in our pursuit of advanced degrees. Learning new things allows us to expand our minds rather than settle or limit our options. It is an empowering experience to become equipped with knowledge. Following that constant urge to do more research, whether it's about health and fitness or uncovering every detail related to your own medical condition, is a good thing.

Gathering diagnostic data, reading scientific studies, or discovering the latest nutraceutical or therapy that might provide symptom relief means you are not solely relying on a doctor to tell you how to feel better.

While the pursuit of external knowledge seemingly moves you forward, you can also become addicted to information gathering. You can become so obsessed with finding an answer to what ails you, or your child, that you simply embody the mantra "I can't give up!" You brand yourself as a "warrior," and you're off and running. Soon you become so disoriented in your hypersaturated environment that you end up going in circles, which further distracts you from looking inside. Hope is a powerful motivator when you're struggling to overcome illness or facing other challenges in life; it is not, however, a strategy. This is an important distinction.

Hope can fuel you to research information that leads to life-changing solutions. Believe me, I wouldn't be where I am today without hope and a passion for research! But obsessively searching for the answers outside of you can be limiting. While I was reading every bit of research on how to reduce pain and inflammation, I was also turning my attention within and looking for the answers that were deep inside me, that couldn't be found anywhere else.

Research in the absence of self-reflection can lead to overwhelm. This can cause higher levels of stress. Your body has built-in mechanisms to help regulate internal stress, which means your body could actually block answers to questions you seek to resolve in the face of complex illness. If your body and mind are overtaxed but you continue to push too hard, you may inhibit the answers from arising naturally in their own due time. For example, under stress your body is in a fight-or-flight response that forces your brain to secrete two hormones, cortisol and adrenaline. This causes you to feel anxious and alert, which would be good if you were in danger and needed to physically react—but in this situation, in which you need to heal, anxiety can prevent you from accessing your inner wisdom. Your inner wisdom is more easily heard in a calm state of flow, where you would be more inclined to think clearly and solve problems. The adrenaline-fueled fight-or-flight response takes precedence over all other bodily functions. This can be particularly challenging if you are the type of person who likes to have all the answers up front, but you are in a chronic state of stress and don't have the mental state to cope and think clearly.

Self-knowledge is different from proclaiming to be an expert on your illness, or the various protocols used for treatment, or even the specific biomarkers associated with a disease that you have been labeled with. Concrete medical information is very helpful and can provide important diagnostic data points—so it's important to get this information and understand it when it is presented by a healthcare provider. That said, medical tests and research data may offer little insight into *why* your body behaves the way it does. No matter what stage of health you find yourself in, you must be willing to ask yourself an important question:

How did I get to this point in my life?

This will often uncover the ways you have compensated for the areas of your life where you might be weak or vulnerable. You can then uncover how you have been compensating and forming patterns around these weaknesses. Once this is clear, you can begin to shift your life to avoid repeating patterns that lead to negative outcomes.

Here are some examples of how this might show up: The lymphatic system is a vital part of our immune system that includes bone marrow, spleen, tonsils, thymus, lymph nodes, and lymphatic vessels. Its primary function is to transport fluid containing infection-fighting white blood cells throughout the body. The lymphatic system also cleanses every cell and organ in the body, providing a pathway for the removal of toxins. Rarely, if ever, do we discuss our lymphatic systems with our doctors. Most of us don't even know how to care for it. Unlike our circulatory system, it has no pump, so it depends solely on the movement of the body for it to flow.

Our sedentary lifestyle leads to lymphatic congestion, or stagnation. Lymphatic congestion is most often brought on by poor diet, stress, environmental chemical exposure, hormone imbalance, and even aging. This is different from lymphedema, which occurs in an arm or leg following cancer treatment when lymph nodes have been removed during surgery.

When stagnation occurs, this puts a stress on the body and the immune system, which often leads to poor health and chronic disease. One of the most common complaints of anyone struggling with lymphatic issues is fatigue. Sadly, with little awareness of the connection to the lymphatic system, the fatigue is usually dealt with in other ways. It may be improperly blamed on poor sleep, thyroid issues, or other hormonal imbalances. In most case, people often self-medicate with coffee, sugar, energy drinks, and alcohol. If you are experiencing lymph-related symptoms, like brain fog, fatigue, itchy skin, consider simple practices that get the lymph moving. Exercise; hydration; and red-staining foods, like cherries, beets, pomegranates, and cranberries, work best.

Unfortunately, we see a similar compensating pattern play out in digestive health. In the United States, up to 70 million people are afflicted with digestive diseases. Heartburn and gastroesophageal reflux disease (GERD) are two of the most common conditions—over 40 percent of Americans have heartburn at least once a month, and up to 35 percent have reflux. Most sufferers and their physicians look to acid-blocking drugs known as proton pump inhibitors (PPIs)—like Nexium, Prilosec, and Prevacid—to mask the root cause of their heartburn symptoms. But we need stomach acid in order to digest our food and absorb nutrients. Reducing the acid in the stomach could have serious long-term consequences, like mineral and vitamin deficiencies. Most people don't know this when they agree to the medication for symptom relief.

If you've been taking acid blockers for many years, you might experience a zinc deficiency or a B12 deficiency that may lead to depression. Sadly, these drugs are now being linked to serious side effects, including Alzheimer's disease, osteoporosis, many different types of infections; disruption of the microbiome, and multiple nutrient deficiencies. It is well established that most people take PPIs for decades, despite their intended purpose as a prescription for short-term use.

Chronic stress affects the nerves in your stomach, making it impossible to process the food properly. It's not uncommon for people to have episodes of reflux during difficult times in their lives. In fact, in order to digest your food well, you have to relax. You also deplete levels of magnesium in your body during times of stress. Magnesium is needed to relax the sphincter at the bottom of your stomach that actually lets the food go down. When you don't have enough magnesium, the food and/or acid could go up and irritate the esophagus. Food sensitivities that may go undetected or undiagnosed by your physician are often linked to heartburn and GERD.

Plus, shifts in your microbiome are common triggers, so a single round of antibiotics or hormone medications, like birth control, prior to the onset of digestive symptoms could indicate that the shift in bacteria may be the cause. A specific bacterium that is often harmless in small amounts, *Helicobacter pylori (H. pylori)*, can be linked to reflux when it becomes too abundant. Once this imbalance is in place, sugar and processed food in the diet can suddenly feed bacteria that should not be in high amounts, thus causing symptoms of reflux.

As you can see, for ailments like reflux and fatigue, the root cause requires self-reflection. They are generally linked to something you are eating, lifestyle factors, medications, or a stressful event. With that in mind, you can resist the urge to suppress it and instead listen to your body and its wisdom.

Of course, not all ailments are so straightforward or so obviously connected to physical symptoms like reflux, but self-inquiry is often more important than the impulse to suppress or cure the actual symptoms. When you stop to reflect on life events that happened at the beginning stages of any dysfunction that may have served as triggers for certain symptoms, you can begin to uncover what your symptoms mean for you. Most people are motivated by the solutions to their problems—that is, symptom relief—but when you are drawn to the *questions*, you stay humble as a student of life. You become your own health detective. You learn about who you are versus becoming solely focused on fixing the isolated issue at hand.

Why am I prone to certain physical symptoms? Where does chronic disease show up in my body? Where am I most vulnerable? What areas do I need to strengthen? This insatiable curiosity will keep you open to new ways of approaching health and resiliency in all areas of your life. Taking the time to notice imbalance before you act on the urge to suppress the discomfort will prevent the root cause of chronic disease from taking hold under the surface.

Life has a funny way of teaching us lessons. When there is something you need to learn, something that you need to work on, the same situation or ailment will continue to resurface until you find a healthy way of dealing with the root cause.

The wisdom of your body should not be underestimated as your most valuable messenger. No one knows you better than you. You are your own healer.

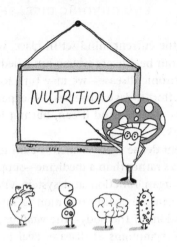

NOURISHMENT

Food Is Information

We are complex organisms, and the cells in our bodies literally get information from everything around us, most significantly from the food we eat. In recent years, the famous quote attributed to Hippocrates, "Let food be thy medicine and medicine be thy food," has transformed into the widely used phrase "food is medicine." As a nutrition educator, this should make me rejoice. Instead, it makes me cringe. Here's why: the quality of our food has changed, dramatically, and for the worse. Food of the lowest quality may lead to chronic disease. And that's exactly what's happening.

With the current mind-set in place, when we fall ill and when our healthcare system has failed us—as it often does for chronic disease—we may turn to nutrition in a last-ditch effort to save ourselves. We expect food to "fix" our chronic disease. And it can, but not in the way you might think.

Nutrient-dense food—which is akin to a *strengthener of weaknesses* rather than a medicine—supports and nourishes our organ function and system vitality. In other words, we can use quality nutrition to support the intellectual wisdom of the body—the *vital force*—rather than oppose the symptoms of disease. Real food is information and has the capacity to communicate to the complex networks in our bodies and initiate healing when it perceives our bodies' unique needs. Our food is coded for our survival.

While quality food certainly has medicinal properties, first we must distinguish that which can be viewed as medicine and that which may be detrimental to our health. Sadly, not all food is created equal. Nutrient-dense foods are real, unprocessed foods that include micronutrients, like essential vitamins, trace minerals, and electrolytes; plus macronutrients, including carbohydrates, proteins, and different types of healthy fats. As humans transitioned from hunter-gatherers to farmers, ranchers, and urbanites, our diets shifted to include more highly processed foods and refined sugars. How we produce food is adversely affecting food quality, both the phytochemical richness of our herbs, spices, fruits, and vegetables and the biochemical richness of meat, dairy, and eggs, as well as the nutritional value of our grains.

The universal notion "everything in moderation" is also woefully out of date. Perhaps it made sense when the majority of people ate whole, nutrient-dense food and chronic disease was not the norm, but today more than 150 million people in America suffer from chronic disease. Author Michael Pollan points out that there are 80,000 known edible plant foods, about 3,000 of which are commonly used in the human diet. And yet over 60 percent of caloric intake worldwide consists of just four highly subsidized and heavily sprayed industrialized crops: wheat, corn, soy, and rice.

In our modern world, where processed food, rancid vegetable oils, high-fructose corn syrup, and artificial colors and preservatives line the shelves of every grocery store, the application of this "go with the flow" attitude comes with great risk. Many individuals acknowledge the value of unprocessed, organic, nutrient-rich foods for a variety of health reasons, however it's still rare to see people fully devoted to a diet composed of them. Access, cost, and social inconvenience are the factors that are most commonly cited as barriers.

To further complicate matters, it seems like every day that another study comes out showing the health benefits of an isolated vitamin, mineral, or antioxidant in the prevention of a certain diseases. Most supplements and nutraceuticals on the market undermine the synergistic effects that nature provides when you consume food in its whole form. Rarely do we discuss that supplementing isolated nutrients can be harmful. Beta-carotene pills, for example, may actually increase cancer risk, as opposed to the whole carrot, which may lower your risk. Collectively, research on isolated nutrients sends a strong message to the public that experts still underestimate the power of whole nutrition and the infinite biochemical data of natural foods to heal and sustain our bodies.

More than 100,000 disease-preventing nutrients known as *phytonutrients* can be found in plant-based foods. From *phyto,* the Greek word for "plant," phytonutrients form a plant's immune system. They increase the plant's ability to survive in nature. What's good for the plant appears to be good for you too. Blueberries contain anthocyanins, which have been shown to improve memory. Tomatoes are rich in the red pigment lycopene, which, according to research, targets heart disease and cancer; and ginger has gingerols that help reduce hypertension. Intake of citrus has been associated with reduced stroke risk, perhaps due to its phytonutrient hesperidin, which has been shown to increase blood flow throughout the body, including to the brain. And before you are tempted to reach for the latest supplement, keep in mind that, when it comes to phytonutrients, the whole food is often greater than the sum of its parts. Taking supplements can support a healthy diet, but it will not correct a poor diet. It's the combination of nutrients working together in conjunction with quality food that keeps us healthy.

Even the health of livestock is enhanced when they forage on phytochemically rich landscapes versus consuming chemically treated, high-grain rations in feedlots.

Of course, our food is more than vitamins, minerals, and phytonutrients; and it's more than protein, fat, and carbohydrates. Food—real food, that is—nourishes the health of your inner ecology by feeding your microbes and communicating with your cells via microRNA-carrying exosomes. A growing body of research on how plants use exosomes as a form of communication is opening up.

Let me explain: Small encapsulated particles from plants, or exosome-like nanoparticles (ELNs), contain plant RNA that is released during digestion and then incorporated into our gut bacteria, which influence RNA expression. A mouse experiment in 2013 used grape-derived ELNs that penetrated the rodents' intestinal lining and stimulated a biochemical pathway known as Wnt/-catenin, which induced intestinal stem cells to protect the mice from developing ulcerative colitis. These results are especially encouraging because these botanical exosomes were capable of modulating unique biochemical pathways for anti-inflammatory responses as well as those crucial to the prevention of autoimmune reactions. These ELNs are not limited to grapes; they have been isolated from foods, including carrot, grapefruit, and ginger root.

According to research led by Dr. Yun Teng, Ph.D., in 2018, ginger ELNs are preferably taken up by Lactobacillaceae and contain microRNA's that target various genes in Lactobacillus Rhamnosus (LGG), including gut barrier function improvement.

The idea that plants communicate for survival is not new. Exosomes may have originally evolved in plants as a means of communication between plant cells and as a way of modulating the first-line immune defenses that plants deploy upon pathogen invasion. Plants are vibrationally sensitive and can respond to sounds in nature, as well as being capable of "learning" behaviors based on repeated stimuli in their surroundings. For example, the sound caused by caterpillars chewing on leaves results in the release of volatile chemicals that repel caterpillars from eating some plants. Plants have also been shown to communicate with other plants in order to defend themselves against predators. Studies have shown that when attacked, plants can "cry for help" by producing chemical signals that attract carnivorous predators of the attacking herbivores.

It turns out that when we eat plants, the same biochemical changes that occur as a result of the plants' survival behaviors become part of our own biochemistry. The genes from the plant are transferred to us through a process called *horizontal gene transfer*, which then affects our microbes and our health. Exchanging epigenetic information with the food we eat is a true testament to how profoundly interconnected we are with nature.

What's exciting is that we are learning more and more about the many ways that the foods we eat every day may exert synergistic effects in course-correcting our gut biology. And perhaps now we can appreciate that when these exosomes are liberated from the foods we eat, they may also serve as a means through which our digestive tract communicates directly with the external environment—a form of cross-species communication.

These food-derived exosomes also support the notion that the value of fruits and vegetables extends far beyond their vitamin, mineral, and bioactive phytonutrient content. What science is beginning to shed light on is that there are subtle workings in the body that we are only just beginning to understand, and that we are a direct extension of our environment. It's a subtle play between our microbiology and genes and the effects of our environment on our genes.

In the same way that your sense of touch delivers information from your environment to the brain and nervous system, your sense of taste also carries strong impressions from the food you eat into your internal environment. The health and vitality of your body, nourished emotions, and resilience are also thought to be correlated with a variety of tastes that are harmonious—or what we might call *sattvic*, an Ayurvedic term denoting a class of foods that are light, fresh, and nourishing. A resilient lifestyle intimately connects you to the natural world through eating and tasting your food with loving awareness. Meanwhile, this awareness is encoded with a nutritional intelligence that Mother Nature has perfectly designed for you.

Taste and smell—the chemical senses—were the first senses to evolve. While taste, as you might imagine, starts on the tongue, there are taste receptors all over the body. Bitter receptors extend far beyond the mouth, lining the esophagus, stomach, intestine, liver, pancreas, and gallbladder, as well as the respiratory and nasal tracts. These widespread receptors trigger a system-wide reaction throughout the digestive tract. Scientists believe that when we are exposed to potentially harmful bacteria and viruses, certain bitter tastes are activated in our mouths and noses, which launches an immune response in the respiratory system.

Bitter herbs have been used for centuries in many different cultures around the world as a digestive aid and even a primer by triggering production of the body's endogenous digestive enzymes and secretion of bile. In essence, they send the signal, "Let's get going; there's work to be done; let's fire it up."

Within the small intestine, we also have specialized cells called L cells that are identical to the bitter taste receptors on the tongue. The lower digestive system is also "tasting" our food, and in this case, when the bitter taste gets exposed to the L cells, it causes them to secrete GLP-1, or glucagon-like peptide 1, into the bloodstream. This secretion stimulates the action of insulin release, helping to control blood sugar levels after eating. In short, the bitter-tasting foods help manage blood sugar and insulin levels. Bitters stimulate all digestive secretions: saliva, acids, enzymes, hormones, and bile. Each of these acts as a solvent to break down our food for absorption, and the quantity and quality of these fluids ensures proper nutrition. Inadequate production of these secretions may be implicated in a number of nutrient deficiencies. For example, inadequate stomach acid will prevent the uptake of minerals, which will in turn rob the body of essential nutrition. Low stomach acid also weakens stomach tissues and is often the foundational cause of esophageal reflux (though esophageal reflux disorders are mistakenly believed to be caused by too much stomach acid).

Why are spices used? The obvious answer is that they enhance food flavor, color, and palatability. People often eat less of foods that provide more sensory pleasure than they do of a blander version of the same foods. The flavor feedback loop occurs when our cells and our microbes respond to the primary and secondary compounds in the spices. Another reason for spice use lies in the protective effects of phytochemicals against the plant's environmental enemies—bacteria and fungi. After all, bacteria and fungi also attack meat and other food items; indeed, some of our most common foodborne pathogens are the same species that afflict living plants. Throughout recorded history, foodborne bacteria have been linked to serious health concerns. However, spices can kill such microorganisms and inhibit their growth before they produce toxins, so the use of spices—garlic, onion, allspice, oregano, and thyme ranking in the top five—reduces foodborne illnesses and food poisoning.

And the wisdom communicated from the food to our bodies does not stop there. When your body is under chronic stress, your adrenal glands produce more stress hormones, and your need for salt increases—hence the cravings for salty foods. This craving is your body's signal that it requires more trace minerals. Calcium is the most abundant mineral in the body, with 99 percent of it stored in the teeth and bones, where it helps to maintain the integrity of the skeleton. The other one percent is found in the bloodstream and soft tissues, where it plays an important role in several biological processes. Calcium has a synergistic relationship with vitamin D and potassium and an antagonistic relationship with magnesium, phosphorus, sodium, iron, manganese, and zinc. For many bodily processes to function optimally, we must maintain the right balance of vitamins and minerals. A deficiency in one might exacerbate a deficiency in another, and when nutrients are antagonistic, they may negatively impact absorption of each other at high doses.

Sourness makes us salivate, which dilutes the chemicals in our mouths and reduces the acidity of sour foods. Sour foods, like kimchi, pickles, lemons, and kumquats, come with all types of benefits: improving gut health, strengthening the immune system, and boosting energy levels.

An estimated three billion people from both developed and developing nations have specific nutrient deficiencies. In the developing world, the results of poor nutrition are deadly: low birth weight, high rates of infection, diarrhea, and other conditions brought on by malnutrition take the lives of millions of people every year, especially young children. In the U.S. and other developed countries, poor nutrition results in higher rates of infection, increased risks of all types of cancer, and an increased risk of obesity. This strain on our health, our economy, and our happiness is real. Nutrient density—or nutritional information—is often reflected in taste and aroma, not the volume and visual aesthetics of our food. When you believe food is information and it's communicating with your body, you realize that taste is not only one of the most pleasurable of the five senses but a surprisingly complex and vital sense that we have yet to fully appreciate. In fact, flavor compounds that make food taste delicious are synthesized from important nutrients, like omega-3 fatty acids and essential amino acids, that make it nutritious. Put simply, food that keeps us healthy and helps us combat chronic disease tastes better.

While the organic movement has successfully reduced chemical residues on our produce and resulted in more environmentally sustainable farming practices, you cannot successfully address nutrient density merely by consuming foods that are organic. Studies consistently show large and very significant variations in nutrients related to other factors, particularly the quality of the soil the plants are grown in. Tomatoes can have up to tenfold variation in Vitamin A from samples collected across the U.S., as well as variations in lycopene, antioxidants, and phenolic and ascorbic acids. In other words, a tomato is not a tomato is not a tomato—even if it's organic. The nutrient density of any plant relies on the soil it is grown in, the water and air that surround it, the original seed it was sprouted from, and how long it sits before it is used.

Sadly, most of the research on taste is devoted to how scientists can manipulate our taste buds to sell us more processed foods. We've all heard about the magical manipulations of fat, salt, and sugar to hook us on manufactured foods. Sure, salt is salty and sugar is sweet. Is there really a difference between pure maple syrup and pancake syrup? Yes, actually, there is quite a bit of difference in how our body interprets sap that runs naturally out of a tree every spring versus a sugary liquid made primarily of high-fructose corn syrup and artificial flavors and coloring.

Even the touted Mayo Clinic issued a report that pancake syrup made from high-fructose corn syrup was essentially the same as pure maple syrup. Real, pure maple syrup contains many different antioxidants in the form of phenolic compounds that are beneficial for reducing free radical damage, which can cause inflammation and contribute to the formation of various chronic diseases. There is evidence from the global scientific community that pure maple syrup contains certain bioactive compounds that help protect the body's immune system and potentially have a positive impact on several areas affected by chronic inflammation. These include metabolism, brain and liver health, and maple's emerging link to a healthy gut.

It also has significant levels of manganese and zinc and has ten times more calcium than honey. University of Rhode Island researcher Navindra Seeram has discovered 34 new beneficial compounds in pure maple syrup and confirmed that 20 compounds discovered last year in preliminary research play a key role in human health, including fighting diabetes. Imagine the irony of finding a potential antidiabetes compound in a natural sweetener!

There is evidence from the global scientific community that maple syrup contains certain bioactive compounds that help protect the body's immune system and potentially have a positive impact on several areas affected by chronic inflammation. These include metabolism, brain and liver health, and maple's emerging link to a healthy gut.

It's possible that our affinity for foods that are naturally sweet may have evolved to ensure the acceptance of sweet-tasting foods such as breast milk and vitamin-rich fruits. There is some interesting research that suggests that we may crave sweets for their pain-reducing properties. Again, these are all signs of our body's innate intelligence and ability to communicate with our food in an effort to help us thrive.

We are complex organisms. We were never designed to live on the limited information from four monocrops that get processed into food-like substances and packaged for long shelf life. We were designed to be part of an intricately complex planet that is remarkably capable of keeping us healthy and in balance.

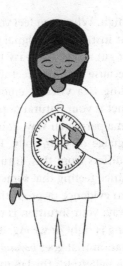

INTUITION

Self-Trust Is My Most Powerful Guide

The power of knowing, that *inner voice*, is not a gift given magically to a select few. It is an ability that you can harness for yourself, and it is your sacred gift. While your rational mind and logical thinking often take center stage, as predictability tends to feel more comfortable, ideally the mind should serve your intuition, or your subconscious.

We've all been told before, "Listen to your gut" or "Follow your heart." These are different ways of saying, "Listen to your intuition." Gut sensations are more common when stakes are high. When you feel you have something great to lose, your instincts will signal you are in danger, and in turn, your gut reacts. It is easy to confuse instinct with intuition because you *can* "feel it in your gut." Literally, a gut feeling is a visceral emotional reaction to something. Instinct is your natural or primal tendency to behave or react in a particular way. Your instincts are the unconscious language of your body. Pure intuition, on the other hand, differs from this. Intuition is when you have the unexplained feeling that something is true, even when you have no evidence or proof that that's the case. Think of it this way: your intuition is the *inner voice* that tells you something is right or wrong. It's subliminal processing of information that goes *beyond* rational thinking or emotion-driven beliefs; it's the language of the soul.

Because healing is a natural process that comes from *within* rather than originating from an external source or treatment, tuning in to intuition as a driver is almost logical. The notion of self-healing is rooted in the understanding of v*is medicatrix naturae,* meaning the body's natural ability to heal. You do not need to understand human biology to appreciate that an intrinsic healing potential lies within you. You do, however, need to trust yourself to cultivate your intuitive energy. Healing is not passive, but this does not mean that you need to be constantly "fixing" the physical body. You must learn how to develop a sense of inner trust, which has been eroded by a culture that gravitates to technological and scientific solutions for almost every problem. If you view your body and your life as constant do-it-yourself repair projects that necessitate counseling, coaching, energy work, cleansing, fixing, and rebuilding, then you are likely chasing a "cure" rather than honoring the natural healing process that can unfold.

There is a difference between curing and healing. Curing relies on an external process, treatment, medication, or intervention. While therapies and interventions aimed at curing may rid your body of specific symptoms, a healing response might not actually take place as a result. Healing, on the other hand, is a restoration of wholeness. So when you rely on treatments from an "expert" rather than saying "I don't know; let me tune in to figure this out," you miss opportunities for a deeper understanding.

Don't mistake this to mean that you should avoid therapy, coaching, or any other support that keeps you strong or that helps you tune in to your body. And, of course, intuition is not a replacement for medical care. Instead, use it to improve your decision-making by adding to good judgment, not replacing it. However, you need to make sure that you are not overdosing on interventions as a way to avoid certain questions that only you can answer. At times you may need to allow the internal healing process to take place by providing an introspective environment that includes periods of rest, pause, and redirection.

Seek healers and practitioners who engage you in the process of tuning in and who acknowledge the power of your intuitive guidance. Our culture considers intuition and the language of the body inferior to intellect. Alternative treatments like energy medicine, homeopathy, acupuncture, and chiropractic modalities, which aim to nudge the body's own healing power, are still underappreciated. Even when well studied, well documented, and considered highly effective, they are often ignored or are considered "probably not harmful" at best by most conventionally trained medical doctors. In addition to the physiological and biochemical shifts in the body to support healing, many of these treatments can help you to harness your intuition by reconnecting you to the source of your symptoms.

All of your experiences provide an opportunity to gather intuitive information about yourself. You may even be surprised that the stronger your intuition becomes, the more clarity you have about other practical choices, like selecting your healthcare practitioners—or, as I like to say, your wellness team. Your model of care may switch to one in which your primary care team is centered around health versus disease, and your "alternative" care providers are for emergency visits only, should you break a bone.

I recall the first resurfacing of my own intuition. Intellectually, I was in the midst of exploring the connection between the microbiome, nutrition, and chronic diseases. But in a quiet moment when the kids were asleep, I was sitting in front of the fire, reflecting on the state of my health, when I was overcome with a sensation I had never had before. My husband was sitting close by, watching a basketball game on TV, when I asked him if he had ever experienced a "burning feeling" in his belly, which I went on to describe as a deep urge or calling. As a sports enthusiast, he immediately compared it to nerves before a big all-star game, which I dismissed as something very different. At the time, I wasn't sure what to call it. I knew what it wasn't—it was not pain, discomfort, or heat. But it definitely was originating in my core. Almost a decade later, I can identify it as my intuition tugging at my attention.

It was a life-changing moment that altered the trajectory of my healing. In its wake, I gained a sense of certainty of being on the right path, which was both unprovoked and undeniable. In that moment, I had a new perception without any expectations.

After that day, I encountered several other experiences and people who deepened my connection with my self-trust surrounding healing, such as the legendary energy healer Donna Eden. Experiencing Donna's energy medicine at her live event was certainly another one of those unique moments that allowed me to move my attention inward toward my energy systems. She taught me that our energy systems have evolved in resonance with our anatomy and our environment over millions of years. But let me be clear, you are not required to enlist any special tools or practitioners to access your own intuition. You just need to learn how to more effectively recognize your energy and, if desired, optimize therapies to assist you with self-healing. This starts by believing in yourself. Learning to recognize the trustworthy voice of intuition over anxiety, fear, and wishful thinking is a major step in "just knowing" what's best for you.

Learning to trust your body again takes time. When you feel your body has failed you, it can be difficult to decipher when something is wrong or when things are simply changing. Initially it can help to think of it as a tool to move you forward and understand yourself better.

Whether you call it a gut feeling, an inner voice, or even a sixth sense, intuition can play a real part in your decision-making. For the first time, researchers at the University of New South Wales in Australia have discovered that intuition does, indeed, exist and that they can measure it. They found evidence that people can use their intuition to make faster, more accurate, and more confident decisions, and published their findings in the journal *Psychological Science*. *Intuition* generally refers to a brain process that gives people the ability to make decisions without the use of analytical reasoning. Despite widespread acceptance of this idea by psychologists and the public, scientists have lacked a reliable test to gather objective data on intuition or even prove its existence.

Previous studies didn't actually measure intuition, because researchers didn't really know how to quantify it. The researchers defined intuition as the influence of "nonconscious emotional information" from the body or the brain, such as an instinctual feeling or sensation. The results showed that when the participants were shown positive subliminal images, they did better on certain tasks: they were more accurate in determining which way the dots were moving. They also responded more quickly and reported feeling more confident in their choice. Participants became better at using their intuition over time. It's all about learning to use unconscious information in your brain. This study also revealed that you can become more adept at trusting your intuition when you use it more frequently over time.

So keep in mind, everything you perceive—everything you sense, or feel, or remember—basically, everything you notice has meaning. Everything is a sign. The language of intuition is not always clear, so tune in and take notice. Nurture what you already know to be true, and build on that process of self-trust to guide you to optimal health.

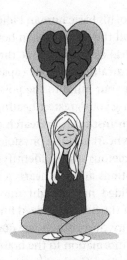

EMOTIONS

*Positive Feelings Recondition
the Mind and Body to Heal*

Every time we have a thought or feeling, it is expressed biochemically through changes in our network of hormones, neurotransmitters, cells, and glands. In short, the body doesn't lie. Our thoughts and beliefs affect our physical condition just as our physical condition impacts our mood. Much as the vagus nerve serves as a superhighway for the microbes between the gut and brain, our emotions also facilitate bidirectional communication between our body and mind. The mind-body connection is not New

Age mumbo jumbo; it's basic human biology, and tapping into it may make all the difference on how well we heal.

Perhaps you feel skeptical about the role that emotions play in your health and your capacity to heal, but it's worth opening your mind to the possibility that your emotions may house your greatest healing potential.

The HeartMath Institute, a research center dedicated to the study of the heart and the physiology of emotions, has conducted numerous studies identifying the relationship between emotions and the heart. A number of their studies have provided new insight into understanding how the activity of the heart is indeed linked to our emotions and our vitality. Surprisingly, we now know that the heart sends more information to the brain than the brain sends to the heart. And the brain responds to the heart in many important ways. For example, as you experience feelings like anger, frustration, anxiety, or insecurity, your heart rhythm patterns become more erratic. These erratic patterns are sent to the emotional centers in the brain, which recognize them as negative or stressful. These signals create the actual feelings you experience in the heart area of the body. The erratic heart rhythms also block our ability to think clearly.

With today's technology we can predict, with about 75 percent accuracy, what someone is feeling just by looking at the beat-to-beat activity. Heart rate variability (HRV) measures the variations in the beat-to-beat intervals by the heart as a response to environmental and psychological challenges. It can measure the flexibility of the heart and nervous system, as well as our capacity to adapt to our mental and emotional states. Research shows that having moderate levels of variability makes us more resilient in life, as we are better able to adapt to life's challenges. In contrast, a low heart rate variability is an indicator of compromised health in the general population.

Researchers have also discovered information encoded within the heart's beat-to-beat intervals by looking at the spaces between the heartbeats in HRV readings rather than the spikes related to the beats themselves. The intervals between the beats are complex transmissions of information used to relay communication between the brain and the body. The autonomic nervous system regulates very important systems in our body, including heart and respiration rate and digestion. The autonomic nervous system has a parasympathetic (rest) branch and a sympathetic (activation) branch. Heart rate variability is an indicator that both branches are properly functioning.

A healthy heartbeat contains healthy irregularities. That's right: even if your heart rate is, say, 60 beats per minute, that doesn't mean that your heart beats once every second—or at one-second intervals, like a clock. Rather, there is variation among the intervals between your heartbeats. The interval between successive heartbeats might be 0.85 seconds in one case and 1.35 seconds in another, for example.

Dr. Joe Dispenza has conducted fascinating research on heart coherence, or physiological coherence, which refers to the heart's rhythms that appear as smooth, ordered, and sine-wave-like patterns. His research suggests each of us is capable of achieving, increasing, and maintaining our heart coherence through the intentional self-generation of positive feelings such as compassion, care, love, and other renewing types of emotions. In contrast, heart incoherence (or imbalance in the sympathetic and parasympathetic nervous systems) is brought on by stress, anger, fear, and anxiety.

In my clinical practice, it was not uncommon for people to come to me asking for nutrition advice to resolve a long list of chronic symptoms they had had for decades. After a thorough health history and careful review of their diet and lifestyle, I'd make some slight adjustments to their diet, but often it was clear that they were on the right track—eating an organic, whole food diet, exercising regularly, sleeping well, and practicing gratitude. What was *not* happening was the emotional unpacking of their illness. Like me, they had experienced trauma and years of failed medical interventions that had led to the end of a successful career, crushed dreams, and in some cases indescribable physical and emotional pain and suffering. So much of their suffering was manifested in their physical bodies—locked up in their muscles and tissues. The musculoskeletal system is the body's interconnected system of nerves, muscles, and bones. The fascia is a layer of connective tissue that weaves through your entire body. It encases your muscles, joints, and bones like a piece of plastic wrap that encircles your whole inner body. The fascia actually holds on to our emotional memory of traumatic events, even if time has passed and we are no longer directly involved in the traumatic situation.

The idea that tissues may possess some sort of memory is a controversial topic in medicine, calling for more research and clinical exploration. But many bodyworkers, at some point in their practice, have experienced phenomena that could be interpreted as a "release" of memory when they have worked on dysfunctional tissues or a source of injury in some individuals. This feeling is sometimes accompanied by some type of sensory experience for the patient, in which an early traumatic experience may be recalled.

Today, more than 100 million Americans suffer from chronic pain. Tissue is not mindless. Thus, touch or manual therapy may "unload" the tissue, causing a change in neural input to the brain, which may trigger the memory. So, as you release fascia, you are waking up the body's sensations and memories of past experiences, which include the emotions that are tied to them.

After my failed back surgery that left me disabled, I turned to myofascial release therapy with the intention of getting some pain relief, increasing range of motion in my pelvis, and helping with restrictions that were affecting my gait. My therapist provided several hands-on techniques that involved applying gentle, sustained pressure to the fascial connective tissue, which did provide improvements in my mobility, but what I did not anticipate was the number of times that I experienced spontaneous and profound surges in my emotions during therapy. It didn't take long for me to figure out that underneath my fascia, I was holding on to patterns of repressed emotional trauma.

When events happen in our life, we experience biochemical changes. Emotions also help us to make sense of our experiences. If you were to receive a cancer diagnosis, for example, you might experience the emotion of fear. Or you might feel anger, sadness, or even determination. Whatever thoughts or emotions you might have, you will also experience a notable physical response: the stress response. Your heart will beat faster, your palms might sweat, blood flow will begin to move toward your muscles and away from your stomach, and your breathing will change and likely become more rapid. Your thoughts, emotions, and sensations all show up as biochemical events.

And guess what? Even if you eventually overcome your illness, the memory of that fear or anger can produce the same response. Biochemical responses are the same whether they are generated by an actual physical event or the thought of one. In a study at Stanford University Medical School, patients who had suffered one heart attack were asked to recount incidents that made them mad. As they did so, the pumping efficiency of their hearts dropped by as much as seven percentage points—a range cardiologists regard as a sign of myocardial ischemia, or low blood flow to the heart.

All thoughts are units of mental energy, or electrical impulses, in the body. So when you harbor negative emotions, you also carry anger, fear, rage, resentment, and even revenge. Even when you think of a person or an incident and there is a negative emotional charge associated with that thought, you are blocking your ability to heal and live your full potential.

Emotions create signals that are communicated through your nervous system on a constant basis. Every cell in your body is in constant communication with each other. For instance, adrenaline (epinephrine), a hormone and neurotransmitter, is associated with the emotional counterparts of fear (fight, flight, or freeze responses). When you encounter, or even imagine, a fearful situation you instantly send an emotional signal to your adrenal glands, which in turn instructs your cellular DNA to code for proteins that combine into adrenaline in rapid succession. Adrenaline enters the bloodstream and increases your heart rate and blood pressure, as well as diverting blood supply from your gastrointestinal tract to the large muscle groups, getting you ready for fight or flight. The bidirectional nature of your emotions and your body's associated physical reactions provides you with a potentially powerful opportunity for self-healing. You can, in fact, begin to release emotions associated with unhealthy molecules and instead foster healthy emotional signals that support your self-healing abilities and help you thrive. It's also important to remember that the experience of intense emotions or stress is not harmful to your health, provided these emotions are expressed and let go of appropriately.

A meta-analysis (results from 101 smaller studies were combined statistically into one single study of several thousand men and women) confirmed that long-term exposure to perturbing emotions is bad for our health. People who experienced longer periods of sadness and pessimism, chronic anxiety, unremitting tension, or increased hostility were found to have double the risk for disease, including asthma, headaches, arthritis, peptic ulcers, and heart disease. Stressful emotions create a chain reaction in the body—stress hormone levels increase, blood vessels constrict, blood pressure rises, and the immune system is weakened. If you consistently experience these emotions, it can put a strain on the heart and other organs and eventually lead to serious health problems.

Emotional intelligence, a term that defines our ability to recognize, understand, and manage our own emotions as well as navigate social complexities, was created by researchers Peter Salovey and John D. Mayer, and later popularized by Daniel Goleman in his book of the same name. While emotional intelligence speaks to our competencies around self-awareness and social relationships, the research into emotional intelligence has revealed some interesting physiological details of how each emotion prepares our bodies for different responses. For example, anxiety is connected to the onset of illness and the slow response to recovery. In the case of fear, the emotional centers of the brain trigger the release of hormones that prepare the body for threat, making us feel edgy and agitated. In response to love, the body is in a parasympathetic pattern dubbed the "relaxation response," one that often facilitates cooperation. Anger seems to be the one emotion that does the most harm, at least when it comes to the heart.

Modern science shows that the health benefits of forgiveness are numerous: better immune function, longer lifespan, lowered blood pressure, improved cardiovascular health, and fewer feelings of anger or hurt. With the benefits of "letting go" so compelling, imagine what can happen if you intentionally choose positive emotions. For example, you can create a positive physiological effect by choosing love or by choosing to heal, an act of self-love. You have been conditioned to think that you cannot control your body. You can in fact set into motion a cascade of at least 1,400 biochemical changes in the body that promote growth and repair through an elevated sense of well-being in a safe environment. Your emotions are extremely important in determining whether you have symptoms of illness or vitality.

Just like a drum beating, your heart has the power to set into motion a sound wave that radiates throughout the body. When you live in the state of gratitude, joy, or love for life, the heart begins to beat more coherently. It appears that the feeling of appreciation is one of the most concrete and easiest positive emotions for individuals to self-generate and sustain for longer periods. The heart has a magnetic field, and this field has an energy. This energy carries a message to the body in response to your emotions. When you shift your attention to feelings of appreciation you change your energy; and this can profoundly change your life for the better.

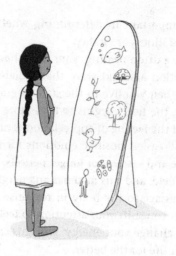

CONNECTION

The Health of Each Is Bound by the Health of All

The medical establishment operates in a way that fosters the idea that each mechanism, organ, and system of the body operates independently. Through this lens, the conventional medical practices that we've all become accustomed to focus primarily on targeting disease in one particular area of the body rather than promoting wellness throughout the *entire* body. The current medical system is largely made up of specialists who are uniquely trained to treat a certain system or part of the body by identifying the seemingly isolated disease, writing a prescription for a pharmaceutical drug, or performing a surgery to correct or, in many cases, remove the damaged body part. This is an isolating, disjointed lens through which to see the body.

Seeing the patient as a collection of separate parts rather than a cohesive, integrated system that is always seeking balance and homeostasis will, more often than not, lead to more disease, more disability, and more suffering. While an acute-care model is effective for infectious disease control or emergencies such as injuries, it's becoming blatantly clear that this model has limitations and is not effectively addressing today's current chronic disease crisis.

When we look at the human body as an interconnected network of vital communication pathways, we understand that everything is connected. A breakdown in one system—immune, cardiovascular, endocrine, digestive, and so forth—will adversely affect the health of the others. Conversely, improvement in one system will positively impact the others. And when there is damage or disease in one organ, the entire body is impacted.

When we draw an analogy between the human body and our planetary ecosystem, we can also imagine how the forests and deserts, meadows and mountains, lakes and oceans, glaciers and rivers, and everything on the planet all rely on one another in order for life to endure and evolve. Similarly, we can assume that each living species (including microbes and viruses) has been perfectly designed and positioned in a way that enables it to receive, metabolize, and transmit information for the benefit of the entire web of life.

Sadly, humans are not honoring the whole. In particular, how we currently produce our food threatens this web of life. In the last 40 years, farming practices have changed dramatically. We now produce a nutrient-deprived food system that has been massively scaled to feed the majority of the developed world with a staple of crops—like soy and corn—that lack medicinal value.

Have you ever driven down a country road, stumbling upon miles and miles of corn or soy fields? That's a monoculture system, where farmers plant a lot of one type of crop. It's devoid of biodiversity; the soil and surrounding environment are devoid of microbes. This kind of industrialized monoculture agriculture is detrimental to the soil; harmful to nature, especially our precious pollinators like bees and butterflies; and counterproductive to human health. It's not working for the planet or our health—yet this is how most of our food is grown.

Because crop loss is a major issue in agriculture due to natural pests and weeds that may reduce yields when they get out of control, the biotech industry has manufactured genetically modified versions of corn and soy crops in an effort to solve this problem. By splicing a toxin-producing gene into its seeds, Monsanto (now Bayer) created crops that "resist" its herbicide Roundup, which contains a highly toxic chemical called glyphosate that kills just about everything in its path. These crops are called Roundup Ready. When farmers plant these crops, they can spray Roundup all over the field to kill the weeds without killing the crop itself. But this remedy was solely focused on problems—the weeds and the pests—with little regard for the whole, including the soil and its microbes, the plants and animals on the farm and in nature, and us, the people who eat the crops sprayed with this toxic pesticide. The pesticide does not wash off; glyphosate residues are found in the vast majority of commercial nonorganic foods.

Mother Nature also responded to this "solution" by developing resistance to the toxins in genetically modified corn. Nature is designed to change and evolve in order to keep up with the environment. So as resistance increases, in order to maintain the promised increased yield (which Monsanto failed to do), farmers must apply more and more chemical pesticides and herbicides to crops. This is expensive for farmers, terrible for the environment, and dangerous for consumers. We now have "superweeds" and "superbugs" that Roundup can no longer eradicate.

More importantly, by their very design, genetically modified organisms (GMOs) are not meant to be more prolific than traditional crops. In other words, they do not increase yields by the seeds themselves producing more numerous, stronger, or healthier plants. Instead, the increase is supposed to be due to lowered crop loss. This is a reductionist approach to agriculture that has had devastating implications on human health as well. Glyphosate, the active ingredient used in Roundup herbicide, is used on both GMO crops and conventional crops in the final stages of harvest. Recently, Friends of the Earth tested for residues of pesticides and herbicides on conventionally grown oat cereals, pinto beans, apples, applesauce, and spinach from national chains like Walmart, Kroger, Costco, and Albertsons/Safeway. One hundred percent of the oat cereal and pinto bean samples tested positive for glyphosate residue. These levels exceed the cancer risk benchmark dose for children stated by the Environmental Working Group by over 2 times (oat cereal) and 4.5 times (pinto beans).

Regenerative agriculture, on the other hand, describes farming and grazing practices that, in addition to food-production benefits, reverse climate change by rebuilding soil organic matter and restoring degraded soil biodiversity—resulting in carbon drawdown and improving the water cycle. Regenerative agriculture treats the land more holistically, taking into account the long-term effects of farming. Experts in regenerative agriculture have proven that when hooved animals (such as cattle, buffalo, and pigs) graze freely on spacious, wide-open fields of wild grasses, their manure fertilizes the grasses so much that it actually sequesters carbon. This type of integrative livestock management is vastly different from CAFOs—concentrated animal feed operations—where animals are packed into cages, knee-deep in dung, and forced to eat GMO grain and alfalfa. This way of raising livestock contributes to the increase in carbon emissions, contaminates the ground and waterways, and produces meat and dairy products that are chock-full of glyphosate residues—and often many other unhealthy chemicals, including hormones and antibiotics.

It's true that most people would likely favor an end to high-carbon, polluting, unethical, intensive forms of grain-fed meat production. But I think, for most people who have concerns for the environment, animal welfare, and personal health, it's not quite as simple to consider just giving up meat as the solution. A critical lesson I've learned as a nutrition practitioner and educator is that we can, and do, thrive on different diets. We cannot, however, thrive on an unhealthy planet. Unless we are sourcing all our products specifically from organic, no-till systems, we are still actively participating in the destruction of soil biota, engaging in a system that deprives other species—including small mammals, birds, reptiles, butterflies, and bees—of the conditions for optimal life. Our ecology is complex, so there's a huge responsibility and opportunity here for all of us to investigate the solutions holistically

With 7.5 billion people on the planet and growing, it's critical to consider all the ways our choices impact our environment. Surely, an increased demand for meat has the potential to increase greenhouse gas emission (GHGE) with unsustainable agricultural practices. Other researchers contend that regenerative agriculture can reduce GHGE and sequester greenhouse gasses, with added benefits that include enhanced biodiversity and ecological function when we rectify damaged soil with plant cover and animal manure. When we consider other factors—like assuring that the diets of lambs include wild plants such as angelica, common fumitory, shepherd's purse, and bird's-foot trefoil because they contain fumaric acid—emissions of methane are significantly reduced.

So perhaps it's not a question of vegan versus paleo, raw versus macrobiotic, or any other superiority of one dietary system over another but rather a question of how we go about producing the food in *any* diet.

It can seem overwhelming, I know, especially when you're dealing with a chronic health issue as I was. Like many people, you may feel it's too much to address such questions as how we grow our food or how we run our healthcare system—but no matter how much or how little each of us gets involved with the "issues," we are *all* part of the web of life. The choices you make—no matter how big or how seemingly small—affect all the other organisms on this planet.

When we come together to address these issues, the challenge we face is not in our ability to become engaged on these topics but instead in our capacity to do so without attachment to our opinions or judgment of others. This is important.

While our dietary preferences are unique to us, the quality of our food choices—that is to say, where our food comes from, what farming practices we support, and the health of our soil, air, and water—is a common thread we all share. As eaters, we are all connected to the future of this planet.

Time spent fighting with each other about one universal way for humans to eat keeps us from achieving what we all want the most: a healthy planet. It would behoove us all to learn more about major environmental issues of our time. The World Economic Forum's Global Risks Report in 2018 identified our most pressing threats over the next ten years, including extreme weather events and natural disasters, failure of climate change mitigation and adaptation, water crises, biodiversity loss, and air and soil pollution.

Arguing over who is right or wrong pulls us away from discussing and, more importantly, implementing all of the possible solutions for a healthy planet for ourselves and future generations. Striving for outcomes that only align with our personal opinions or preferences while condemning others who don't share our dietary preferences creates social division. The future of food should not be vegan versus carnivore but rather a food system that honors and respects the lives of animals, plants, microorganisms, and people versus a system that demoralizes, dehumanizes, and destroys our biological commons.

We all have the opportunity to exemplify our personal choices in the way we live our lives, which often includes educating others, but we need to avoid the temptation to condemn those who oppose our views or have different dietary preferences. We can take a position on important topics knowing that all good causes lead to the same place. There is never just one way to solve a complex problem.

And please don't misinterpret this shift in mind-set as a call to stay quiet. Our need for connection and unity *requires* us to speak up. We must never miss the opportunity to speak our truth, nor should we stay silent and let others—politicians, our neighbors, the "experts"—dictate what we should do for important matters of planetary or human health. Instead, I'm suggesting we share our views and remain open to hear the insights from others—opening our hearts and our minds to the common thread that unites us all: healing. With nature as our teacher, we can co-create with her, acknowledging and supporting her agency.

We are here to grow and leave this earth a better place. We can only do that when we learn from each other. We need to be able to flesh out our ideas and thoughts—letting go of our urge to win the debate. As we enter the discussion with curiosity and respect for everyone at the table, and leave our judgment at the door, we can work together to heal ourselves and the planet.

Ultimately, environmentally destructive behavior is the result of a failure to recognize that human beings are an inseparable part of nature and that we cannot damage it without severely damaging ourselves. Everything we do to the earth we are doing to ourselves. We are part of the earth.

Everything in nature follows a code of interdependent communication. If we want to survive, we're going to need to learn this way of communicating as well. Separatism is indeed at the root of disharmony. Conversations on meaningful subjects with people we know and love, or with people we have just met, create ways to belong and in turn can help ease the pain of loneliness, particularly when we approach them with curiosity rather than judgment. Social isolation has been shown to set off a cellular chain reaction that increases inflammation and suppresses our bodies' immune response to disease. Research has also shown that having weak social ties can be as harmful as smoking and twice as harmful as being obese. Think about that for a minute—loneliness can make you sick!

Even brief moments of conversation can rescue us from loneliness and isolation—reconnecting us to the web of human thought. Our relationships shape us, and supportive relationships create security and health in our lives. Living your life with an emphasis on direct ways of connecting with others, which includes engaging with eye contact, facial expressions, tone of voice, posture, gestures, or touch, may reclaim a part of your deep social self and allow you to become more fulfilled in your life. I believe we all have come to a better understanding of where our debate and division can and cannot take us, and many people are ready to reclaim real connections again. The good news is that we have everything we need to start—we have each other.

Part II

BEHAVIORS

Health is a gift you give yourself. It is acquired through your daily habits—your behaviors. The quality of your health emerges out of your habits and the consistency by which you apply them. By exploring the set of beliefs that shape your views about healing from chronic disease, you can embody that state of mind through your actions.

Behavior that is incongruent with your values rarely creates optimal health. You may want to heal, but if don't believe you hold the power, it will be hard to change the behaviors that led to disease in the first place. On the other hand, if you believe healing is possible but fail to take consistent action, you may not get very far either.

Assuming you are ready to build a new foundation with the shift in mind-set from Part I, the power of behaviors is really the application of a more intentional way of living by leveraging healthy, yet practical, habits in your daily life. With the right knowledge and strategies, healing and achieving resilience should feel attainable. Lasting change is deeply rooted in your behaviors. Every action you take is casting a vote for the life you want.

Keep in mind, these lifestyle behaviors are not meant to control any of your existing *bad* habits. I believe that when your primary motivation for change is to break bad habits, then you feel forced to *move away from* something that is impacting your life negatively. While swapping out bad behaviors for seemingly good ones may be beneficial, I have found that when life gets tough, it's not uncommon to slip back into our old ways. However, if your initial focus and intention are on building the life that you want, then your intention is to *move toward* more beneficial patterns.

In this book, we will be focusing on this action of *moving toward* healthy behaviors with the added benefit of impacting the ecology and diversity of your microbiome, which is one of the key drivers in achieving optimal health and long-term resiliency. All lifestyle behaviors influence the microbial diversity, or lack thereof, of your microbiome.

Microbes are the origins of all life on our planet, silent allies to our evolution and our health. You will learn more about our bacteria and the role they play in supporting our health in Part III of this book. For now, I will focus on the actions that you can take every day that will shift your inner terrain in your favor. Let's go.

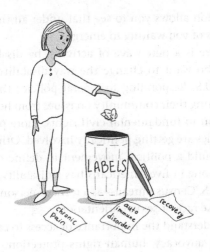

DROP THE DISEASE LABELS

Dr. Wayne Dyer once said, "Any time you start a sentence with *I am*, you are creating what you are and what you want to be." Learning to set clear boundaries around your illness or disease allows you to find pockets of joy, which gives you a window in which to seek healing and refuge. Resilient people understand that there is a separation between who they are at their core and the cause of their suffering. Illness or disease might play a part in their story, but it does not overrule their identity. This distinction allows you to see that under all the suffering are parts of you waiting to emerge.

There is a new wave of activism by disabled Americans who want to change the way disability is viewed in the U.S. Responding to federal policies they feel are threatening their community on issues from healthcare to education to fundamental civil rights, more people with disabilities are getting politically involved. Others are trying to build a political movement to define disability— roughly one in five Americans has a disability, according to the U.S. Census Bureau—as a form of personal identity, much like race or sexual orientation.

I understand the importance of access to care and the need for advocacy, human rights protection, public service, and connection to the larger collective group for the greater good. During one of the most difficult and sickest times of my life, I chose to volunteer on the board of directors for a nonprofit organization in my community that serves over 40,000 people with special healthcare needs. I was in the depth of my own medical crisis and was labeled "permanently disabled for life" at the young age of 35. In the midst of saying good-bye to a corporate career that I loved and in the most painful time in my life, I also had to resist the urge to *become* my label while taking a stand for individual rights and advocacy across all areas of health and education.

Admittedly, at times I did find myself getting attached to my disease label, which subtly goaded me into seeking quick fixes, cleanses, supplements, medications, and cures to "undo" my label. In some ways, the label served as my "get out of jail free" card for the days I simply couldn't cope. It validated my suffering, and it also allowed me to qualify for medical services. In this way it became very difficult for me to separate from my illness. Consciously choosing not to identify who you are with your disease is complicated. To foster a life of what's possible *in spite of* the cards you were dealt takes practice, support, and great courage.

Disease labels distract even the most well-meaning practitioners. Protocols begin to dictate the direction of care, and your ability to listen to the language of your body becomes foggy again as you become attracted to the idea of streamlining the healing process. Becoming your "label" can lead to a loss of self, and this inevitably leads to a weakened state. Ideally, the focus needs to be on restoring health.

Let me be clear: I am *in no way* suggesting that we minimize anyone's suffering, including our own, or avoid getting to the root cause of any illness by clearly naming it, explaining it, and having a clear therapeutic plan. In fact, with improved communication, less judgment, and personalized care, people are much more likely to improve. But the statistics and prognoses for people with chronic disease are alarming.

Six in 10 adults in the United States have a chronic disease. Four in 10 have two or more. According to the Centers for Disease Control and Prevention, chronic disease is the leading cause of death and disability in the United States, accounting for 70 percent of all deaths. The Center for Managing Chronic Disease at the University of Michigan states that chronic diseases are long-lasting conditions that usually can be controlled but not cured.

They go on to explain that people living with chronic illnesses often must "manage" daily symptoms that affect their quality of life, and experience acute health problems and complications that can shorten their life expectancy. That's true. And until we all have the courage to talk about what's really causing this problem, we will keep managing and treating the symptoms.

You are not to blame for your illness. But in order to *truly* heal, you must be willing to accept what comes your way and honor these experiences as messages. If you feel victimized, you will miss the opportunity to witness the power and wisdom of innate healing. Feeling victimized only adds to your illness. Once it becomes a consistent part of your daily actions, it can, and often will, qualify as an illness in itself.

Let's reframe it so you understand what I know to be true: chronic disease is preventable and reversible. That means if you don't have a chronic disease, you can avoid getting one. And if, like millions of other Americans, you do have one, or more than one, you can reverse it. Perhaps you now know what I mean by the difference between *healing* and *curing* that I wrote about in Part I. You are your own healer. The wisdom lies within.

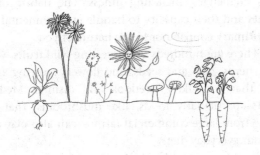

EAT ON THE WILD SIDE

If you think kale, turmeric, and blueberries are the only superfoods available today, you are missing many of nature's original heroes and their inherent resilience-boosting qualities. Wild plants—including some you may easily recognize, like dandelion, broadleaf plantain, stinging nettle, red clover, spearmint, burdock, and wild ginger—embody the knowledge of how to survive in all conditions, even the most inhospitable. Plants can't fight off their enemies or even hide from them in nature; instead, they produce chemical compounds as a form of protection against insects, disease, preying animals, and the damaging effects of ultraviolet light and inclement weather. And by extension, when we consume them, wild plants contribute to our capacity to survive and overcome life's challenges, including illness. The nature of wild plants and their capacity to handle environmental stress is a primary contributor to the nature of you.

There are hundreds of interesting wild fruits, vegetables, herbs, nuts and seeds, and flowers growing around you that you likely overlook and dismiss. Medicinal foods—particularly foods, like mushrooms, that don't come from large commercial farms—can also play a part in your everyday diet.

Reishi is considered the "queen of mushrooms" because of its reputation for revitalizing the whole body. Used in traditional Chinese medicine for at least 2,000 years, it is one of the most widely researched mushrooms thanks to its ability to boost the immune system against pathogens, bacteria, and parasites. Its triterpenes improve circulation, which leads to better mental clarity and improved physical appearance.

Dandelions, the prolific wild "weed," are also well adapted to the world of disturbed habitats that we live in. The plague of urban lawns across the world, their deep, meandering roots usually break as they're pulled out of the ground, leaving behind pieces that will regenerate into new plants. They can fertilize themselves and disperse seeds as early as a day after the ubiquitous yellow flower opens. Dandelions have eight times more antioxidants, two times more calcium, three times more vitamin A, and five times more vitamin K and vitamin E compared to spinach. They resemble two other edible species of the early spring and late fall: chicory and wild lettuce.

Our modern diets tend to habituate us to foods heavy in sugar, salt, and fat, so we often lack a taste for the bitterness that occurs in many wild edible greens. Extreme bitterness is, of course, unpalatable and can indicate the presence of toxins. There are, however, many shades of bitterness. Developing our ability to appreciate them can help expand our palates beyond the sweet, oily, and salty foods that too often define what is tasty. Calcium is bitter. Historically, hunter-gatherers consumed more calcium-rich wild greens and had much stronger bones to show for it. Their diet, like that of the last remaining hunter-gatherer tribe, called Hadza, consisted almost entirely of food they found in the forest, including wild berries, fiber-rich tubers, honey, and wild meat.

A recent study in the journal *Science* focused on the Hadza, who reside near Lake Eyasi in the central Rift Valley of Tanzania, Africa. They basically eat no processed food—or even food that comes from farms. The researchers analyzed 350 stool samples from Hadza people taken over the course of about a year. They then compared the bacteria found in the Hadza with those found in 17 other cultures around the world, including other hunter-gatherers. During the wet season—when Hadza eat more berries and honey—they have a greater variety of microbes. During the dry season, Hadza eat a lot of more meat—kind of like Westerners do. And their microbiomes shifted as their diet changed. Some of the bacterial species that had been prevalent when their wild, fiber-rich food intake was higher disappeared to undetectable levels, similar to what's been observed in Westerners' guts. The good news is that these missing microbes returned, indicating that the microbiome is plastic, depending on diet.

Adding more locally grown greens to your diet is one of the simplest ways to eat on the wild side. Growing your own food at home makes sense—homegrown fruits, vegetables, and herbs are fresher, more nutritious, and better tasting than store-bought, conventionally grown fruits, vegetables, and herbs. But more important, you have the advantage of producing food that is clean and naturally organic—free from genetic modification, chemical pesticides, fertilizers, herbicides, and pesticides.

Plants may also lose nutritional value when they are stored for lengthy periods, or when they are being transported over long distances. The most nutritious greens are the ones that are dark in color. Dark varieties indicate a higher level of a phytonutrient called lutein, which is a potent antioxidant that will protect you against inflammation. Another factor to keep in mind is that plants need sunlight to grow and produce carbohydrates but also must protect themselves from the damaging UV rays by manufacturing their own botanical sunscreen. Because most of its leaves are exposed to the sun, loose-leaf lettuce must produce extra phytonutrients. When you eat this lettuce, you become a beneficiary of the plant's self-defense system—the plant's protection becomes *your* protection against cancer, cardiovascular disease, and inflammation. Conversely, the leaves sheltered on the inside of the tightly packed iceberg lettuce have one percent of the antioxidant activity compared to the sun-exposed leaves on the outside of the plant.

Home food production also connects you with the seasons and the cycles of nature. Local food and foraged ingredients allow you to choose flavors reminiscent of the current season, like eating a juicy heirloom tomato at its peak or picking black raspberries during the early summer.

Our early ancestors foraged and collected a variety of edible wild plants as a way to survive. However, whereas everyone knows what a tomato, a squash, and a pepper look like, most of us never learned which wild plants are edible, except perhaps a few fruits and berries. Fortunately, there are a variety of foraging guides available today to help beginners get started on the journey of learning how to identify some of the most common wild edible plants that can be found growing in and around your environment. Always consider the importance of properly educating yourself before consuming wild plants on your own. Though they are rare, there are wild plants toxic enough to kill you, so take your time when foraging, and work with a trained guide. There is an app called Flower Checker where you simply snap a picture of a wild plant with your phone and for the cost of one dollar per submission you are connected to a team of live, international botany experts that can identify the plant for you within 24 hours.

And when it comes to eating wild foods, don't overlook wild fish, like mackerel, sardines, salmon, and anchovies. A study at the University of New York at Albany found that the environmental pollutant dioxin is 11 times higher in farm-raised salmon than in wild salmon. Dioxins are highly toxic carcinogens that are stored for a long time in your body. Their half-life in fat cells is 7 to 11 years. They are known to impair the endocrine, immune, nervous, and reproductive systems. Wild-caught salmon is very high in omega-3 fatty acids, as well as selenium, niacin, vitamin B12, magnesium, and vitamin B6.

You can begin by incorporating foods like wild blueberries, which are rich in phytonutrients and easy to find in every local grocery store. Farmers' markets are also great for seasonal finds like yellow dock, wild radish, elderberry, wild mushrooms, and a variety of wild berries.

As the idea of eating more food produced locally grows in popularity, a logical extension to obtaining food from farmers markets is turning to nature's garden, the wild edible plants that can be grown in your own backyard. Gardening—in any form—is one of simplest ways you can invest in your well-being. Start small: sprouting microgreens, a potted herb garden, a small raised bed of vegetables, or a single fruit tree.

The good news: you can't go wrong. Wild foods and foods grown in home gardens tend to be a good source of phytonutrients and prebiotics—food for your gut bacteria (which you will learn more about in Part III). For now, you can relish knowing that prebiotics—like those found in wild foods and plants—may be more potent than any store-bought probiotic in terms of shifting the microbial composition of your gut as they stimulate your gut bacteria. Plus, the time we spend outside harvesting our food in the garden, foraging for wild foods, or simply expanding our diets by trying new foods is good for our overall health.

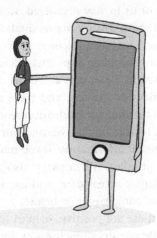

MASTER YOUR
ATTENTION

There's an invisible problem that is profoundly affecting the health of everyone in society: competition for our attention. We now have the ability to fill every waking moment with distraction. We can label it "work," "entertainment," "efficiency," even "connection," but we intuitively know that being perpetually plugged into our technology is unhealthy.

Like most people, you probably think of technology as simplifying your life—*saving*, not *stealing*, your time. With digital tools like maps, calendars, and ride-sharing apps like Lyft and Uber, modern technology has made it easier for all of us to stay organized, work from home, and even travel more. Things like meditation apps and fitness trackers can move you closer to your wellness goals. In fact, there are countless apps that allow you to easily monitor your weight, heart rate, and other diagnostic data points at any time of the day, and these same apps are contributing to technological advancements in hospitals. Needless to say, technology has become our go-to method for tracking medical information. If you have health challenges, this is priceless. Technology also allows you to explore new things, access data, and expand your horizons in ways you could never do before.

Certainly, these are positive, helpful ways that technology has made our lives much easier, more organized, and safer, which can reduce our stress and contribute to a healthier, and perhaps better, quality of life. In the examples I've mentioned, you are in fact in charge of *how* and *when* you use the technology. You are the master, if you're diligent.

But if we want to explore all angles of technology, then we must look not only at what it can do *for* us but also at what it does *to* us—our minds, our relationships, and our experiences as human beings—and also the unintended consequences.

Face-to-face conversation has many virtues; it's timeless and our most basic tool. Modern technological advances have created challenges to this: we are always plugging in, yet we have sacrificed conversation for mere connection. The brain has two sides: the social, more emotionally dominant right side of the brain and the literal, logical, and more objective left side. The right hemisphere picks up the subtler signals of someone's inner state—their feelings, meanings, and intentions—but is less likely to be as engaged on digital screens as it is during interactions that happen in person.

Now let's consider the Internet, which began as a way to share information from computer to computer and has since transformed into an endless, multifaceted outlet for human energy and expression—all in the palm of your hand.

Facebook, Twitter, Instagram, and Google have produced amazing products that have benefited the world enormously. But these companies are also caught in a race for your finite attention, of which they need to win in order to make a profit. Constantly forced to outperform their competitors, they must use increasingly persuasive techniques to keep you glued. And it's working. Snapchat, the app that self-destructs messages and photos within 10 seconds, has seen huge growth, with about 150 million photos shared per day.

These companies direct news feeds, content, and notifications at our minds, continually learning (based on our behavior) how to hook us more deeply. Unfortunately, what's best for capturing your attention isn't best for your well-being. We know that you get a hit of dopamine from social media "likes." In times of stress, you may even turn to social media instead of people for comfort. Through your experiences with both Facebook and Instagram, you may even be getting good at "filtering" your experiences so that what you share with others is a limited "highlight reel" of your life.

Why is this important? Because these are not neutral products. They are designed to addict you. This race to keep you on-screen 24/7 makes it harder to disconnect, which in turn increases stress and anxiety and reduces sleep. The use of social media has been likened to a softer version of the numbed state that gamblers get from slot machines—when the money no longer matters, you are just operating "in the zone."

Tristan Harris founded the Center for Humane Technology after spending three years as a Google design ethicist. Called the "closest thing Silicon Valley has to a conscience" by *The Atlantic* magazine, Tristan developed a framework for how technology should "ethically" steer the thoughts and actions of billions of people away from screens. He points out that a select number of technology companies (Facebook, Instagram, and Google) profoundly influence where our attention goes. And these platforms are ultimately designed to please those who pay to keep them in business: the advertisers. So essentially, advertisers are paying for your attention.

The problem with this lies in the fact that humans have vulnerabilities, particularly vulnerability to persuasion. This is especially true of those who are trying to overcome health challenges. With exposure to various elements of digital media, these vulnerabilities can be amplified or even exploited. During my own health crisis, one of the things I struggled with was the lack of clarity on the best treatments, nutritional advice, or supplements for symptom relief. I found myself constantly searching online for answers. This kept me in a constant state of vulnerability to persuasion. I was not making much progress, and instead, I was bouncing from one idea to the next, distracted by a new set of promises or strategies claiming to help me. This isn't to suggest that the Internet can't serve as a valuable resource. However, the design of digital platforms is to make us act impulsively. Every day, you are pulled to act against your better judgment. Computers, not you, get to decide based on your clicks, likes, shares, and views what shows up at the top of your "feed." The things that work best at capturing your attention are not necessarily the things that strengthen your life and make you stronger. And as a result, you are losing your ability to think for yourself.

To be clear, my goal isn't to imply that we cannot achieve resilient health unless we resist the use of technology. Instead, I'm suggesting that we consider the impact it is having on our ability to truly care for ourselves in a way that leads to significant health outcomes. We should consider our return on investment for our time spent online.

Your handheld devices are another piece of the puzzle. According to the latest Internet trend report by Kleiner Perkins Caufield & Byers, people check their phones 150 times a day. It's the new normal. Your precious smartphone could easily be implicated in so many of your current health problems—sleep disturbances, anxiety, stress, neck pain, inability to focus, headaches—heck, it might even be easier to list the things phones *don't* mess with. Sadly, most of us have built our entire daily schedule around the premise that we can always be on—always reachable, always working, always parenting, always available to anyone who might need us. You are trapped in a nonstop chain of events, digitally linked together.

If your goal is to cultivate resilient health, you must recognize the clear distinction between living your life while using digital tools of technology as your servant and allowing them to pull your vital energy from you. They cannot become a distraction from your most valuable assets: *real* people and *real* experiences.

Our devices are doorways into a virtual world that includes a persuasive landscape. How we behave in that space determines our experiences. We must be brave enough to recognize when we have slipped into the addiction to these spaces. Many times, when you move toward your devices and smartphones to get something done, you are actually moving away from something else.

When you reach for your devices, you should get into the habit of asking yourself, *How is this serving me? Is this moving me closer to my goal?*

When you begin to recognize how and when you are using your technology, then you can take back your authority. It doesn't mean you won't take moments of pleasure to watch a funny video, or read an article for pleasure, or scroll through photos to catch up on everyone's "first day of school" photos. It does mean that *you* decide when you want to carve out that time. *You* decide how to use your time and attention.

Time spent on devices is time *not* spent actively exploring the world and relating to other human beings—in other words, cultivating health. After all, when it comes to getting *back* time wasted online, I'm afraid there is no app for that.

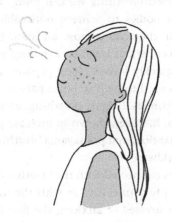

LEARN TO
BREATHE

Take in a deep breath. Feel the wave of oxygen, nitrogen, and carbon dioxide pass over your ribcage and swell your lungs. Now let it go. Before consciously inhaling, you probably weren't thinking about how you breathe at all. The respiratory system is somewhat unique among our body's systems in that we are both its passenger and driver. We have the luxury of letting our autonomic nervous system do the work, or we can decide to override the rhythm of our breath.

With controlled breathing we can nudge other systems within our bodies to achieve noticeable physical effects, although they are almost all short-term. The Valsalva maneuver, which involves exhaling while closing the throat, quickly lowers blood pressure and raises the pulse, and is used to help stabilize patients suffering from heart arrhythmias. Lamaze breathing, used by many pregnant women, has been shown to increase pain tolerance and aid relaxation, and pranayama breathing is practiced in yoga worldwide.

Our ancestors connected with the breath more closely as the breath of life connecting us with the universe. If you've ever been stressed or anxious, the first thing that deserts you is the breath: your chest becomes tight, and as the lack of oxygen increases, a sense of panic sets in. When I think back to times of stress, they were always met with the phrase "just breathe."

The breath moves through our bodies from birth until death, and with so much tied up in our breath—and the simple gift of being able to work with this most potent of autonomic functions—it's worth exploring the benefits of rethinking how we breathe.

Our breath is connected to our emotional state. When we panic or get anxious, our breath becomes shallow and rapid. With each breath, millions of sensory receptors in the respiratory system send signals via the vagus nerve to the brain stem. Fast breathing, or overbreathing, sends signals to the brain at a higher rate, triggering it to activate the *sympathetic* nervous system, which in turn increases stress hormones, heart rate, blood pressure, muscle tension, sweat production, and anxiety. On the other hand, slowing our breath—by breathing through the nose—induces the *parasympathetic* response, dialing down all of the above as it turns up relaxation, calm, and mental clarity. Nasal breathing automatically limits air intake and forces us to slow down. In fact, proper nose breathing imposes more resistance to the air stream than does mouth breathing, resulting in 10–20 percent more oxygen uptake.

When we breathe through our mouths, we bypass many important stages in the breathing process. The nose is a specifically designed organ of our respiratory system that increases circulation, blood oxygen, and carbon dioxide levels; slows the breathing rate; and improves overall lung volumes.

We also know from studies on yoga and meditation that there is a very direct relationship between breath rate, mood state, and autonomic nervous system state. The autonomic nervous system governs the body's responses, dialing functions like heart rate, respiration, and digestion up or down as necessary in response to potential threats. Evolutionarily, this has worked as a survival mechanism, but today's nonstop barrage of smartphone pings, e-mails, and news updates can trip your body's alarms—and often.

Deep breathing, often referred to as belly breathing, has been scientifically shown to lower blood pressure and heart rate, boost brain health and growth, and even change genetic expression by evoking the *relaxation response*.

For many of us, relaxation means zoning out in front of the television or tablet at the end of a stressful day. But this does little to reduce the damaging effects of stress. To effectively condition ourselves to handle life's ebbs and flows, we need to activate the body's natural relaxation response. Discovered and coined by American Institute for Stress founding trustee and fellow Dr. Herbert Benson, the relaxation response is a mentally active process that leaves the body relaxed, calm, and focused. The key, of course, is to breathe properly—through the nose and deep in the belly.

Belly breathing—in conjunction with nasal breathing—is the most efficient way to optimize our health and activate the relaxation response. Many people who breathe through the mouth too much are conditioning themselves to be shallow chest-breathers. The breathing muscle is the diaphragm, which should rise and fall with each breath, producing a belly movement. This movement massages the stomach and vital organs of digestion, promoting good bowel elimination from the body. This type of breathing also stimulates the vagus nerve, a cranial nerve that starts in the brain stem and extends down below the head to the neck, chest, and abdomen, where it interconnects to all the organs of the body to convey sensory information about the state of the body's organs to the central nervous system.

Focused breathing helps us feel connected to our bodies—it brings our awareness away from our worries and quiets our mind. A Harvard study that examined blood samples of individuals before and after their breathing practices showed a post-practice improvement in metabolism and a suppression of genetic pathways linked with inflammation.

Breathing, much like the practice of meditation, is a way of conditioning the body and mind for times of crisis.

It's in the moment of chaos that we will find our greatest need to return to our breathwork for rescue.

Another practice that can be used to enhance relaxation is Khechari Mudra, in which you curl the tongue and connect it to the palate. This creates an energetic circuit of the front and back meridian channels with the intention to strengthen the body and stimulate the meridian connection points associated with our master glands, the pituitary and pineal.

Since we know that chronic inflammation has been linked to diseases such as Alzheimer's, depression, cancer, and heart disease, it's fair to say that better breathing may not only change our lives but also save them.

By using something as seemingly simple and powerful as our breath, we can heal our bodies and minds. When asked what his favorite practice was, the author, monk, and peace activist Thich Nhat Hanh replied:

> *There are people who say that I teach only one thing: breathing in and breathing out. They are right. With mindful breathing, we're more present for ourselves and for the world. It helps us transform the suffering within and to be in touch with the inter-being nature of reality. So we only need to practice mindful breathing— that is enough.*

I agree.

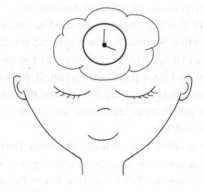

RECLAIM THE POWER OF SLEEP

Six hours or less of sleep a night is the norm. Like me, you probably have read or been told about the benefits of rest—and the risks associated with not getting enough of it. For example, sleep allows you to consolidate and store memories, process your emotional experiences, and replenish glucose (the molecule that fuels the brain). Research shows that sleep deprivation doesn't just lead to poor judgment, lack of self-control, and impaired creativity—it can increase our risk for Alzheimer's disease, cancer, diabetes, depression, obesity, cardiovascular disease, and more.

On top of this, it doesn't take many nights of sleep deprivation to render the body immunologically weak. Dr. Michael Irwin at the University of California, Los Angeles, has performed landmark studies revealing just how quickly a dose of short sleep can affect our ability to fight cancer. Examining healthy young men, Irwin demonstrated that just a single night of four hours of sleep swept away 70 percent of the natural killer cells circulating in the immune system relative to a full eight-hour night of sleep. This is a dramatic state of immune deficiency to find yourself in, and it can happen very quickly—after essentially one "bad night" of sleep. A number of prominent epidemiological studies have already reported that night-shift workers with disruptions to their circadian rhythms have significantly higher odds of developing different forms of cancer. To date, these include associations with prostate cancer, breast cancer, uterine or endometrial cancer, and colon cancer.

Exactly how and why short bouts of sleep may cause cancer is also becoming clear. Part of the problem relates back to the agitating influence of the sympathetic nervous system as it is forced into overdrive by a lack of sleep. Ramping up the body's level of sympathetic nervous activity will provoke an unnecessary and sustained inflammatory response from the immune system. Short spikes of sympathetic nervous system activity that trigger inflammation are not harmful; however, when left switched on, in a *chronic* state, they can manifest as health problems, including those related to cancer.

Inflammatory factors associated with sleep deprivation may also be used to help spread cancer to other territories in the body—a state called *metastasis*, when cancer breaches the original tissue boundary of the origin. Studies on sleep-deprived mice, who suffered a 200 percent increase in the speed and size of cancer growth relative to a well-rested group, demonstrate just how much the lack of sleep can influence the growth of cancer. In the postmortems of the mice, it was also clear that the cancer was even more aggressive in the sleep-deficient animals, spreading to surrounding tissues, organs, and bones.

All species, especially humans, have a biological need for sleep, in which the brain enters a state of inactivity that enables the elimination of beta-amyloid (the waste product that builds up in the brain of Alzheimer's patients). In short, the brain has a method for removing toxic waste that actually ramps up during sleep by pumping cerebral spinal fluid through it and flushing waste back into your body's circulatory system, suggesting this "housecleaning" could even be one of the primary purposes of sleep. Our cerebrospinal fluid circulates up and down the spine and into the brain itself, acting as a cleansing system for the brain and our central nervous system. This incredibly efficient system dumps about three pounds of waste and plaque from the brain via your glymphatic system each year while you sleep. So poor sleep means poor brain waste removal.

Perhaps even more compelling is the most recent connection on how active herpes infections in the brain may accelerate amyloid deposition and the progression of Alzheimer's disease. The research suggests that amyloid, an antimicrobial peptide, is protecting the brain against bacterial and viral infections. Beta-amyloid is a way for the body to trap and permanently sequester invading pathogens, which also gives newer parts of the immune system time to get mobilized.

Dr. Jonathan Kipnis, whose research teams discovered the glymphatic system—the network of lymph surrounding the brain—developed the seventh sense theory: All the senses report directly to the brain, providing intelligence about the workings of the internal and external environments of the body. And all the senses are areas with high concentrations of microbes, which—via the lymph-carrying immune system—communicate critical self-preservation information to the brain. Just as the immune system's major role is to detect populations of pathogenic microbes that may cause harm, as the "seventh sense," the brain's lymphatics are sensing survival threats in the central nervous system.

The two neurologists at Mass General Institute who began this exploration, Robert Moir and Rudolph Tanzi, suspected beta-amyloid is usually good—unless the brain starts making *too* much. Then it can kill brain cells and lead to dementia. They also note that even though we really concentrate on these plaques and tangles in Alzheimer's disease, it looks as if it's the brain's immune system that's gone awry, leading to the question: What's causing the innate immune system to overreact to viruses and bacteria that get into the brain? Or perhaps we are not sleeping enough (my thoughts, not theirs) to effectively cleanse the brain. Until we know more, I'm going to reclaim the power of sleep to give my brain what it deserves—rest.

In addition to this critical role in keeping the body's master computer clean and online, sleep also allows for energy conservation, repair, and growth processes. During the sleep cycle, our hormones enter an anabolic state so the body can produce growth hormones as well as promote the maintenance and repair of muscles, tissues, and bones. As you sleep, the body's immune function is also restored, an effect that in turn can positively affect collagen production, the protein that gives your skin strength and structure.

Insufficient sleep attacks the very physical structure of your genetic material.

The spiral strands of your DNA are tightly wound together into structures called chromosomes. To protect the ends of your chromosomes, you have telomeres, which serve as a cap, if you will (think of the end of shoelace). If your telomeres become damaged, your DNA is vulnerable. Recent studies now reveal that less sleep and poor sleep quality is linked to damaged capstone telomeres of the chromosomes. This damage appears to mimic aging.

In order to turn this knowledge into a lifestyle behavior that is sustainable, you must first understand how your body knows it's time to sleep. One of the big misconceptions about sleep is that melatonin is responsible for generating sleep itself. While melatonin helps regulate the *timing* of when sleep will occur by signaling darkness, it has little to do with activating sleep itself.

Soon after dusk, melatonin is released into the bloodstream from the pineal gland, an area situated deep in the back of your brain. The suprachiasmatic nucleus communicates its repeating signal of day and night to the brain and body by using melatonin as its circulating messenger. Melatonin then corrals the sleep-generating regions of the brain to symbolize the official start time of sleep itself. For this reason, melatonin is not a powerful sleeping aid in and of itself. In fact, once sleep is underway, melatonin slowly decreases in concentration throughout the night and into the morning hours. In the absence of circulating melatonin, which occurs naturally, and as sunlight enters the brain (even through the closed lids of the eyes), the brain is informed that the sleep cycle is over. This allows for the beginning of the wakeful period. The 24-hour circadian rhythm is the first of two factors that determine the wake and sleep cycle; the second is sleep pressure.

With each waking minute, a chemical called adenosine builds up in the brain. It continues to increase in concentration the longer you are awake. The more this chemical accumulates, the more the brain registers the amount of time that has elapsed since you woke in the morning. A consequence of high amounts of adenosine in the brain is an increased desire to sleep. During sleep a mass evacuation is underway as the brain has a chance to remove the day's buildup of adenosine. Surprisingly, the 24-hour circadian rhythm of the suprachiasmatic nucleus and the sleep-pressure signal of adenosine are two distinct and separate signals. Even in the absence of sleep, your circadian rhythm continues to fall and rise on the basis of what of time day or night it is—despite what level of adenosine pressure exists in the brain.

To determine the quality of your sleep, you can start by asking yourself a few important questions after waking up in the morning: *Can I fall back asleep at 11 A.M.?* If the answer is yes, you are likely not getting the sleep quality or the number of hours you require. *Can I function without caffeine?* If the answer is no, you are most likely self-medicating through a state of chronic sleep deprivation. If you didn't set an alarm, would you wake up at the same time every day? Do you have difficulty focusing or remembering simple tasks?

I am by no means offering a comprehensive review of sleep or sleep disorders, of which there are now over 100. Instead I am attempting to engage you in an appreciation for sleep and to reverse your neglect of it. It is vital for all functions of the body but is the least understood and most underutilized tool in the pursuit of wellness, longevity, and healing. And, best of all, it's free!

For now, your most practical and cost-effective tools for improving sleep include lifestyle adjustments that can balance your sleep-wake pattern, such as maximizing light exposure during the day as well as minimizing light (especially blue light from technology) during the night. Stick to a consistent sleep schedule—go to bed and wake at the same time each day. Set the bedtime mood with a cool, dark, tech-free bedroom. Avoid, if possible, medications that disrupt your sleep, including over-the-counter medications for coughs and colds. Reconsider your relationship with stimulants like caffeine and nicotine, avoid alcohol before bedtime (robs you of REM sleep), and avoid heavy or large meals late at night, as they can interfere with sleep. If tracking your sleep cycle interests you, consider a device like the Oura Ring, which is my personal choice.

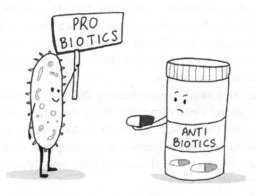

PROTECT YOUR MICROBIAL ALLIES

Microorganisms normally inhabit almost all surfaces of the human body exposed to the environment. Even the intestines, which are exposed to our food, medicine, and anything that enters the body through the mouth, constitute an especially rich and diverse microbial habitat—approximately 800 to 1,000 different bacterial species. We humans are mostly microbes, over 100 trillion of them.

Each year, 47 million unnecessary antibiotic prescriptions are written in U.S. doctors' offices and emergency departments. Many of these unnecessary prescriptions are for bacterial infections that do not always need antibiotics, like ear infections. Many more are for acute respiratory conditions—common colds, sore throats, and bronchitis—commonly caused by viruses, which do not respond to antibiotics. The CDC estimates that at least 50 percent of antibiotic prescriptions for these acute respiratory conditions are unnecessary.

In 2015 alone, approximately 269 million antibiotic prescriptions were dispensed from outpatient pharmacies in the United States, enough for five out of every six people to receive one antibiotic prescription each year. At least 30 percent of these antibiotic prescriptions were unnecessary.

These excess prescriptions each year put patients at needless risk for reactions to drugs or other problems, including *C. difficile* infections. In other words, antibiotics can make you more vulnerable to serious bacterial infections in your normal daily life.

Antibiotics represent an important advancement in modern medicine. Since their discovery in the 1920s, they have allowed us to treat bacterial infections, such as pneumonia and tuberculosis, that might otherwise have been lethal. But antibiotics, for all their effectiveness on "bad bacteria," operate at a cost to the "good bacteria" stored in the gut, which can impact digestion, mood, and overall immune function, among other things.

Last year alone, drug-resistant bacteria, or "superbugs," killed 700,000 people worldwide. Superbugs are projected to be more lethal than cancer by 2050. Dr. Margaret Chan of the World Health Organization has said that we're fast approaching a time when "things as common as strep throat or a child's scratched knee could once again kill." This is largely due to our compromised immune systems. Chronic diseases, cancer, cardiovascular problems, and diabetes are by far the leading causes of premature death in the world, and they are avoidable with a strong immune system.

Because of this, it's important to collaborate with your doctor to avoid unnecessary antibiotic use when creating an effective treatment plan, being mindful to first take care of your microbial partners and protect your gut health in the process.

Besides their direct ecological effects on the composition of our gut microbiota, antibiotics affect the manner in which our microbes regulate our basic physiological processes. This includes the immune system's capacity to fight infections, as antibiotics indirectly alter the effectiveness of both innate and adaptive immune responses.

Inflammation-enhancing alterations in the gut microbiota can be produced by antibiotic exposure and are likely to play a predominant role in metabolic disorders such as obesity, metabolic syndrome, and diabetes.

Of all the locations in the body, the highest numbers of bacteria and other organisms can be found in our digestive tract. It is here that our commensal gut bacteria produce their own antibiotic called *bacteriocin*. Although the role of bacteriocin is not yet fully understood, it is generally accepted that these endogenous antibiotics function to kill off invading pathogens and prevent the overgrowth of unwanted bacteria. They are tools used by our own beneficial flora to keep everything else in check.

When we take prescription antibiotics, we damage these commensal gut bacteria and their protective properties.

It is clear that the excessive, widespread use of antibiotics in our culture has created many threats, including increasing the prevalence of antibiotic-resistant pathogens, which have become a global challenge for infection control. But the effects of excessive antibiotic exposure can be seen not only in pathogenic bacteria but also in the beneficial microbiota of our body.

It is also important to consider the vulnerabilities we create through our consumption of nonorganic foods that are sprayed with glyphosate, a registered antibiotic, and the widespread antibiotics used in the feed of industrialized animals, which we then ingest via the animals' meat. The bacterial imbalances caused by these common indirect antibiotic exposures can negatively affect our health in numerous ways and for long periods of time. When the quality and diversity of our protective microbes decline, pathogens can thrive. Furthermore, all bacteria produce waste, but the metabolic by-products of pathogens are inflammatory, creating messages of systemic, chronic inflammation in the body that underlie many diseases and conditions, such as cardiovascular disease, dementias, bipolar disorders, arthritis, autism, and more.

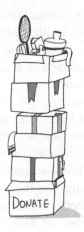

SIMPLIFY

Collect moments, not things. We are constantly pulled toward complex living, but often the most powerful way to nourish our health and open our lives to more abundance is to create space. We can do this by simplifying our day-to-day life and minimizing our tendency to gather material things. This does not mean we can't have nice things or that we are somehow relegated to consignment shopping and repurposing used items in order to live a life of fulfillment. We do this by simplifying our lives. A simple life means different things for each person. For me, it means eliminating all the excess and unnecessary so that only what is essential remains—that is, swapping chaos for peace.

Simplifying is an inherently personal process because what is essential for your home, health, and happiness is different from what is essential for someone else. Recognizing exactly what is most valuable to you allows you to create a life that reflects your values.

In our culture of accumulation, this practice takes time and patience to master (at least for me anyway). My husband and I often joke that we need to invite people to stay with us often so we can be "forced" to straighten up and declutter our home even more—scrambling to clean up before our company arrives and begging our kids to do the same—and we always feel better about our space and the way it makes us feel once we are done. Things stay clear for a while, but the level of clutter eventually begins to creep up again.

If your home is like mine, you might ask yourself the same question as I did: What's the harm? Well, maybe more than you realize. Scientists who study dust say that it not only holds a long memory of the contaminants introduced to the house but also acts as a continued source of exposure. Dust, and the pollutants attached to it, gets resuspended when it's disturbed and will recirculate throughout the house, picking up substances, before returning once more to the floor or surface. According to an environmental chemist at the University of Toronto, even after regular cleaning, dust accretes and may retain legacy pollutants such as DDT that were banned half a century ago.

Other research shows that clutter increases our stress levels. For me personally, it was consuming my time, money, and energy—looking for things that should have been easy to find and purchasing things we already had. Princeton scientists discovered that a cluttered environment limits our ability to focus, and researchers at UCLA discovered a link between high levels of stress hormones and a high volume of household objects.

While most people will be motivated to remove clutter because of its visual nuisance, many will be surprised by how liberating cleaning can be once you recognize that you are also creating abundance by allowing more energetic and mental space in your life. It really does impact the health and well-being of your family in a host of ways you can't even anticipate. It's about preparing an environment where everyone in your family has the best chance to succeed. Your space should include some of your favorite things from your past, but more important, the space in which you live should be open to the person you want to be.

When we are healing, it's important to evaluate our environment. What is the environment we are spending our time in? Is it full of clutter, excess stuff, or things that don't inspire us?

Does it remind us of how we want to feel, or does it reflect how we feel on the days when we feel *stuck* and *heavy*? Oftentimes we set personal health goals but can't get to them because the busyness of life gets in the way. This could be one of the big reasons why you feel you can't make gains.

When I began to apply practices of decluttering (such as the KonMari method) and shifting toward a life of minimalism, I could see that I was gaining more focus, clarity, mastery, and space in my energy field—all of which were helping me to feel healthier and stronger. Sounds strange, I know. But in the past, I had made the mistake of trying to organize my way out of our family clutter. Don't get me wrong, we were not dealing with any level of clutter worthy of an episode on the reality show *Hoarders*, but I would find myself feeling constantly overwhelmed with the daily tasks of sorting through stuff.

Our family of five was putting out a serious volume of laundry, dishes, school paperwork, sports equipment, clothes, and seasonal decorations—it just never seemed to end. And I seemed to be the only one in charge of all the *stuff*. When you focus on "organization," you avoid letting go of things you simply don't need, while feeling like you are making progress because your space is getting neater once again, albeit temporarily. Organizing first means you are making space for things you probably shouldn't keep while ignoring the root of the problem: too much stuff.

Joshua Becker, the founder and editor of Becoming Minimalist—a website that inspires millions around the world to own less and live more—also points out that although a degree of consumption is necessary, limiting your purchases to what you and your family need will help you manage the clutter in your home. As a leading voice in the minimalism lifestyle, he suggests asking yourself these questions before you buy: Do I really need this item? Will I have a place to store this when I get it home? How much extra work will this possession add to my life? Am I buying it for the right reasons? Keep in mind that, while it takes effort to reduce your consumption, at least initially, the choice to do so is laden with meaning.

Consuming less benefits those you might never see, people who bear the environmental impact of our over-consumption. You also have the opportunity to use your extra savings to benefit others. As a bonus, you will be relieved from spending time, money, and energy collecting and maintaining possessions you don't need or use. This leaves more time for you to spend doing what's important to you.

The intention behind this behavior is to get you to declutter, minimize, and simplify your life, but also to fully grasp why this change is needed in your life. By living a life with less, you will find the life you want by getting to the heart of what you need.

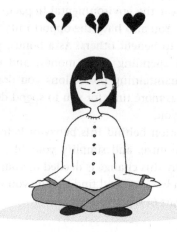

REDEFINE STRESS

Historically, the stress response was essential for our survival, as it still can be today during emergencies. Stimulated adrenals can help you react quickly in the midst of chaos and navigate your way out of dangerous situations. Stress has a reputation for its negative health impact and is largely identified as something to be avoided as much as possible. But stress isn't always a bad thing.

We have been conditioned to think that we can "manage" or "control" our stress, which is often generated from sources outside of our control—like our work, relationships, traffic, politics, death, trauma, and so on. And once we are in a state of stress, we are more likely to engage in unhealthy lifestyle behaviors as a reaction to the overwhelm.

Stress is a stimulus. When we redefine it as such, we can begin to understand that its negative effect on us implies we are losing our ability to cope. Therefore, trying to control or manage it will likely be ineffective and certainly not sustainable. Certainly, using behavioral techniques like daily breathwork during stressful situations can help serve as an anchor, but rather than using lifestyle strategies to merely *navigate* stress, you must build up your capacity to *adapt* to it—and you should start working on this now, long before stress strikes.

Nature teaches us that stress may actually have some positive attributes. Plants increase polyphenols when they are exposed to stressful elements of nature, such as severe weather, disease, or predator attacks. During times of anticipated droughts, plants have the capacity to upregulate polyphenols, which turn on their longevity genes so that the animals that eat the plants can tolerate longer periods without rain. We too benefit from eating plants that are subjected to changing, stressful environments (remember the wild foods!). And there's much to learn from these plants, which are conditioned to respond in kind to all of the elements—good and bad.

Similarly, we can use stress as a stimulus for growth and change. The key is to recognize these opportunities and acknowledge them as life-enhancing rather than debilitating. Since you can't avoid stress or get rid of it altogether, you can *redefine* what stress is for you and recondition your body and mind to respond differently to it. You are an intelligent being with very complex organs and systems that harmonize and function beautifully. You are designed to survive and thrive in a world of challenges. Your capacity to recover and rebound from challenging events, including illness, is stress resilience.

We can transform our response to stress by *defining* it rather than *denying* it. This is not about dwelling upon it but is instead about clearly recognizing the stress we are facing. Research shows that just acknowledging your stress can register proactively in your brain, shifting you from the automatic and reactive centers to the more conscious and deliberate ones. In other words, purposefully acknowledging stress lets you pause your visceral reaction, allowing you to choose a more life-enhancing response. Resilient people understand that stress is a part of living with the ebb and flow of life. As hard as it is in the moment, it's better to come to terms with the truth of a difficult situation or major challenge than to ignore it, repress it, or deny it.

Symptoms of stress and even illness can be signals of poor adaptation, not an end result. When these symptoms continue—that is, when they are chronic—they can begin to change your brain. Chronic daily stress—like being overworked, malnourished, or in unhealthy relationships—can reduce brain size, structure, and function. Stress begins in the hypothalamic-pituitary-adrenal (HPA) axis, a series of responses between the endocrine glands in the brain and in the kidney that control your body's response to stress. When stress is detected, the HPA axis is activated and releases the hormone cortisol to prime the body for action. But elevated cortisol for long periods of time wreaks havoc on the brain, particularly the part of the brain called the amygdala.

As levels of cortisol rise, electric signals in the hippo-campus—the area responsible for learning, memories, and stress control—deteriorate. The hippocampus also inhib-its the activities of the HPA axis, so when it weakens, so does our ability to cope with stress. Chronically elevated cortisol can also cause the brain to shrink, making it hard for us to concentrate. Exercise and meditation increase our ability to handle stress and increase the size of the hippocampus.

The effects of stress don't stop there—they trickle down to our DNA. In landmark studies by Dr. Michael Meaney and researchers at McGill University we saw some of the first clues about how social interactions help to shape our epigenome. They showed that there were dif-ferences in the development of rat pups' response to stress between high- and low-nurtured rats. Mother rats that spend a lot of time licking, grooming, and nursing their pups verses others ignoring their pups play a critical role in how the pups responds to stress later in life. The pups of nurturing moms turned out to be less stressed because their brains developed more cortisol receptors, which stick to cortisol and dampen the stress response. The research-ers also found that the high-licker moms were releasing high levels of serotonin in the offspring, which is a natu-ral antidepressant. The nurturing ultimately changed the epigenetic markers on the rat pups' DNA leading to life-long changes in their stress response.

The pups of negligent moms had the opposite out-come, and became more stressed throughout life, growing up to be aggressive and anxious. They received a message from their mother that something in their environment should make them cautious. This environmental information affects which gene is expressed without directly changing the genetic code. Even more shockingly, the epigenetic changes caused by that one single mother rat were passed down to multiple generations after her. In other words, the effects of that one action were *inherited* and female pups that had high-licker moms became high lickers when they had their own pups. But the researchers made other important discoveries; they switched some of the rats at birth and found that the pups DNA methylation took on the pattern of the foster moms', not their genetic mom's DNA. Taking it one step further, they reversed the DNA methylation patterns after a rat had reached adulthood, eliminating the rat's stress response.

This study is so powerful for a couple of reasons. It showed that a safe, stable, nurturing environment helps develop a healthy stress-response system for adulthood. It showed that the epigenetic code can be reversed. Expressions of genetic patterns that are set up early in life are not fixed. Your genetic code is sensitive to environmental conditions so positive lifestyle choices can shift things in your favor. You can change your body's reaction to different stressors by reconditioning yourself to adapt to stress.

We all seem to agree chronic stress is a major issue contributing to poor health. However, the focus continues to be on managing and controlling it rather than building an adaptive response. Recently, some professional sports have rolled out a new strategy called *load management*, referring to the deliberate reduction of physiological stressors in order to facilitate athletic performance. In theory, this approach sounds similar to our modern-day self-care methods, and it seems simple to apply to life outside the sports arena to help people cope with the stressors of chronic illness. But this can be a slippery slope when it comes to healing from chronic illness and building resilience. Remember, stress is a stimulus and dose matters. However, your response to stress is the litmus test.

Ancient philosophers would likely advise us to periodically embrace suffering as a way to strengthen our resolve and build mental and physical toughness. When we get into the habit of protecting ourselves, rather than conditioning ourselves, we become victims of stress.

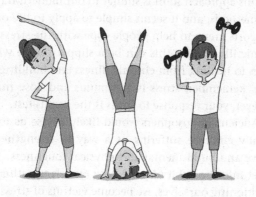

MOVE YOUR BODY OFTEN

For most people, exercise is something that involves special athletic wear, a gym membership, and an extra hour in the day to sweat. Some people love it, but many don't. However, exercise can be structured in a way that does not require us to go to any fitness extremes to undo the damage of being sedentary most of our day. In fact, for most people on the healing path, exercise should really be replaced by functional movements throughout the day and some short-duration, higher-intensity training as tolerated.

Research has shown that even if you exercise daily, if you are sitting at a desk for eight hours a day, you are still at a high risk for cardiovascular disease and other chronic conditions. So the key is not to structure your movement into one single exercise session per day but instead to engage in physical movement all *throughout* your day.

Physical exercise has been shown to have a wide range of positive health effects, such as lower risk of cancer and stroke, better cardiovascular health, stronger muscles, and a greater retention of bone density, which is usually lost as a person ages. It also benefits our mental health by affecting the production levels of a brain protein called *brain-derived neurotrophic factor*, or BDNF for short, which increase after exercise. BDNF has already been shown to enhance mental abilities at the same time as it acts against anxiety and depression. Exercise has numerous neuroprotective and cognitive benefits, especially pertaining to memory and learning-related processes, including hippocampal neurogenesis, the process by which new neurons are formed in the brain. As they say, neurons that fire together wire together.

Movement also gets the blood pumping, primarily because it improves endothelial function. The endothelium is a thin layer of cells that lines the blood vessels. These cells produce nitric oxide, which keeps the blood vessels healthy. Movements that promote nitric oxide production, like resistance training, are essential for overall health because they allow blood, nutrients, and oxygen to travel to every part of your body effectively and efficiently. The blood vessels only store about 90 seconds' worth of nitric oxide before they need to manufacture more, so working each major muscle group for short periods gives us the most efficient workout to tone and build muscles. The body has the ability to regenerate nitric oxide every couple of hours, giving us the opportunity to release it multiple times a day, which means that one effective way to increase muscle function is to incorporate short-duration exercises several times a day.

Aerobic training, such as walking or jogging, hiking, swimming, resistance training, push-ups, weight training, yoga, and sports is a way to infuse movement into your day. The types of movement you choose should be things you enjoy so that you will stick to them in the long term.

Japanese scientist Dr. Izumi Tabata, Ph.D., and a team of researchers from the National Institute of Fitness and Sports in Tokyo were able to demonstrate that only four minutes of high-intensity interval training had much greater impact on both the cardiovascular and musculo-skeletal systems compared to a workout that lasted one hour. The high-intensity workout, called Tabata, is structured to last only four minutes. It works like this: go to your maximum ability for 20 seconds, rest for 10 seconds, and complete 8 rounds. This shows that we do not need to grind away on an elliptical machine at the local gym for an hour to see results. In fact, this is exactly what we *don't* want to be doing.

While doctors used to think that we needed to engage in at least 30 to 60 minutes of exercise a day, current research is finding that we can see benefits with shorter bursts of physical activity. Several high-intensity activities lasting 15 minutes per week, like swimming or weight-training, can kick-start your metabolic rate, reduce body fat, and increase muscle mass. The focus is not on losing weight; it's on living longer and healthier.

Even infusing your day with a variety of movement is beneficial. In a study published in February 2013 in the *American Journal of Health Promotion*, researchers at Oregon State University looked at more than 6,000 American adults and found that even small amounts of physical activity—like walking while talking on the phone—for up to 30 minutes a day can be just as beneficial as longer workout sessions at the gym. The key is to keep moving.

Of course, moderate movement will not result in elite athletic performance, and if you do not modify your routines, you can easily reach a plateau once your body has adapted to a routine. Variety in movement is one way to prevent boredom associated with doing the same activity day after day, and research has also shown that adding variety to an exercise program can improve adherence. We also know that many of the body's physiological systems, like our muscles, adapt to exercise routines within approximately six to eight weeks.

However, there's one caveat, which is that the advantages of adding in variety seem to apply best *only* once you have made a commitment to consistency, which appears to be where many people who are struggling with chronic illness seem to fall short. That is why the focus of this behavior is on moving often. I always say consistency trumps novelty. Once you've mastered good form and consistency, you can build in variety and intensity. In other words, don't be too quick to "mix it up" if that has the potential to get you overwhelmed and make you lose focus.

Creating a routine that you can commit to and see improvements from is an important first step. Consistent movement leads to progress. From there you can build on strength, flexibility, and endurance, which are key attributes of long-term health.

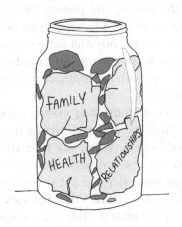

PICK THREE

When facing tough times, especially overcoming illness or disease, we often put our own dreams on hold. It's not uncommon for people to describe their suffering as feeling like they are being pushed by the universe through painful measures as some sort of test in life. If you are stuck and cannot seem to break the cycle of your suffering, then it may be time to consider creating a new vision for your life—one that includes *ikigai*. *Ikigai* is a Japanese concept that means "a reason for being."

Behaviors that make one feel *ikigai* are not actions that we are forced to take, nor are they tied to simple hobbies. Instead, they are linked to living in a way that gives to the next generation. Contributions to raising the children, tending to the garden, and passing down culinary wisdom and traditions are all examples of this. When you live each day intentionally and serve others, you experience a steady, naturally occurring forward motion and are better able to cope with hardships, depression, illness, and life's challenges.

A small act of kindness or sharing advice may seem subtle, but these are powerful factors in your motivation to move forward. When you trust that you live in an abundant universe and allow yourself to give freely, you raise your frequency and put yourself in the flow to receive abundance in return. When you seek ways to serve others, you are suddenly shifting your energy into living, creating, and contributing versus fear and coping—and therefore stepping outside of your own suffering.

So many of us walk through life feeling numb and unsure of how to connect with our "purpose in life." This can be very frustrating, especially if you feel the urge to make a difference in the world, as so many of us do. Be wary if you find yourself in pursuit of a special calling, as you may be missing the opportunity to serve a life with daily intention, which is often the road that leads to your greatest mission in life.

Your worth is not measured by your productivity. Your to-do list is just that: a list you use to remember what you need to accomplish on any given day. It solves the problem of forgetfulness and relieves your worries. It can feel so gratifying to cross items off our to-do lists. But aside from that, it does little to help us actually accomplish anything that is *truly* meaningful.

You might be familiar with the story of a professor and his "Jar of Life." He stood before his class and wordlessly picked up a large, empty mayonnaise jar, which he proceeded to fill with rocks about two inches in diameter. He then asked the students if the jar was full. They agreed that it was full. The professor then picked up a box of pebbles and poured them into the jar. He shook the jar lightly and watched as the pebbles rolled into the open spaces between the rocks. The professor again asked the students if the jar was full, and they asserted that it was indeed full this time. The professor picked up a box of sand and poured it into the jar. The sand filled the remaining open areas of the jar. "Now," said the professor, "I want you to recognize that this jar signifies your life. The rocks are the truly important things, such as family, health, and relationships. If all else was lost and only the rocks remained, your life would still be meaningful. The pebbles are the other things that matter in your life, such as work or school. The sand signifies the remaining 'small stuff' and material possessions. If the sand is put into the jar first, there is no room for the rocks or the pebbles. The same can be applied to our lives. If we spend all our time and energy on the small stuff, we will never have room for the things that are truly important."

This lesson is a valuable one. The challenge, of course, is applying it to our daily life. How can we turn this into a lifestyle habit that optimizes our health and builds resilience?

One of the biggest challenges we all face in our modern world is too much to do with too little time. On top of that, one of the greatest misconceptions is that high achievers are multitaskers. Actually, the research shows that when we do more than one thing at a time, we don't do any one thing well at all. Multitasking gives us the *illusion* that we are accomplishing more in life, but we end up falling short on the things that matter most. While I am certainly in favor of prioritizing our time so that we accomplish more things in less time, I understand time is a precious resource for all of us.

This is especially true, and challenging, when you are trying to overcome illness while at the same time managing other life obligations like work, family, learning, raising children, household chores, and social obligations.

Make a list of all the hats you need to wear—all the relationships in which you need to play a part. And then decide what's important that you can accomplish over the course of the next week. For example, Sunday might take on the focus as a "family day." On Friday, you may carve out time to be with a good friend. Wednesday, you plan school activities and send off an invitation to the school play to the grandparents. It's simply not practical to wear every hat in one day. By shifting your focus to the week, you chunk the time you need to dedicate to obligations accordingly, which will free up the space you need for setting your weekly *top three*.

This is where you will identify the key areas of your life that matter to you the most, choosing just three things that you want to accomplish in that week that fall into any one of the core areas (or large rocks) of your life. This is to move you toward your goal of resilient health by shifting your lifestyle patterns and consciously choosing to set up your plan in "weekly sessions" that target only the things that enrich your family, improve your health, and impact your life in some way—that is, fulfill your *reason for being*. Yes, the other "stuff"—dishes, laundry, work, errands, grocery shopping, meetings, yard work—needs to get done, but remember, those obligations and activities fall in the *pebbles* and *sand* categories. Your goal is to make sure that every week you have at least three simple goals checked off in the "big rocks" category. No matter what!

One goal per week may be fine once in a while if it's big and important. But four or more goals means you're probably putting small or unimportant things on your weekly goal list. Remember, your "pick three" need to fall under the "big rocks" categories of your life.

Pick three is less about productivity, goal setting, or prioritizing your to-do list. It's a behavior that should reframe the way you see and structure your time for the things you care about the most, whether that's spending time with your children, starting a business, taking a class, or writing a book. It's about making the most of your days so they are stacked with the things that matter to you, so your life feels more fulfilling. It's about living with *intention*.

You will inevitably have less time for yourself during some weeks than during others, but even that's no excuse to skip the healthy practice. Instead consider ways to bundle your activities. For example, on days when unexpected events crept in, I knew I was short on time, but I had committed to finishing a meaningful research project and wanted to take advantage of the gorgeous weather, so I took my paperwork outside to the local state park. This allowed me time to squeeze in a brisk walk, catch up on some vitamin D, and finish my project. I could have just as easily stayed in my office and then felt resentful that I had wasted a beautiful day working indoors. Instead I combined my activities and felt accomplished and refreshed. Small wins have a strong positive effect.

When progress happens in small steps, your steady, forward movement toward important goals can make the difference between a great day and a terrible one. The power of progress is a dominant factor in achieving wellness.

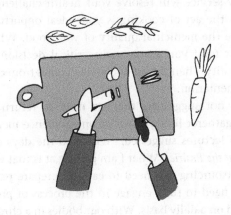

COOK YOUR
OWN FOOD

We have altered our environment so much that our access to "food" requires almost zero effort. We can stop at a store on every corner or drive up to the side of a building and be handed our meals through a window. We can even summon our food with a few swipes of our smartphones. Historically, our ability to eat included hunting, gathering, or harvesting food from our environment. Without effort, we didn't eat.

Cooking has never felt more important for human and planetary health than it does now. While you might even think a few healthy recipes or joining a meal kit delivery service will resolve your health challenges, the truth is the act of cooking is your ideal opportunity to enhance the medicinal quality of your food. When you shop for food you get to make critical decisions about food quality. Then the art of cooking comes from culinary experimentation.

I'm not suggesting that we need to return to our hunter-gatherer lifestyle—or as one audience member at one my lectures suggested, "return to the days of *Little House on the Prairie*." What I am getting at is that we must stop outsourcing our need to eat and prepare real food, and we need to fully engage in the process of preparing our food on a daily basis. With our bodies in a chronically fed but undernourished state, our balance is off.

Cooking puts you in the driver's seat of your health. Once in a while, skip the recipe and focus on stocking your pantry with quality ingredients, and learn basic culinary techniques that will allow you to turn just about anything into a masterpiece using what you have available in the cupboard, refrigerator, and the garden. It takes practice, and mistakes will happen, but eventually you will master a few signature dishes. Start with simple building blocks, like high quality ingredients and employ simple techniques like infusing your olive oil with turmeric, which contains curcumin and has been studied extensively for its benefits in reducing inflammation, arthritis pain, cancer, and stomach, skin, liver, and gallbladder problems, as well as Alzheimer's disease.

Let's face it: nourishing yourself and your family with home-cooked food can feel overwhelming. Without the confidence that comes from knowing how to identify nutrient-dense foods and ways to execute traditional culinary practices, we are left vulnerable to the tempting marketing tactics of the food industry. Certainly, cooking requires forethought, preparation, equipment, and patience. Even so, the results are often superior to food served outside the home.

Chronic disease does not discriminate—50 percent of children the U.S. now suffer from chronic disease. If we want to reverse this trend and give them the opportunity to pursue their dreams instead of a lifetime of disease management, we must change the way we nourish their bodies. We as a species did not evolve to eat frozen chicken nuggets, pinwheel pasta, and cheese sticks wrapped in plastic.

For thousands of years, eating was considered a sacred event. It was understood that the intention and energy put into preparing the food, as well as our frame of mind while we ate—as in, eating with awareness in a relaxed, conscious manner—would deliver superior health benefits. Even the few extra minutes to warm our food on the stovetop builds in a natural, mindful pause that "zapping" our food in a microwave for 30 seconds steals from us. Meals in almost all culinary traditions are conversations chefs have with history and their patrons. In our own homes, we have the opportunity to explore the healing power of food.

My family meets in the kitchen every night to sit down at the table and share a home-cooked meal. I was not taught how to cook growing up; this was something I taught myself when the quality of food and time together became part of our family values. We are building a life for ourselves together around that table. What helps me make cooking our food a priority in my family is keeping it simple. No elaborate recipes, just traditional dishes with lots of flavor.

Time magazine published a piece, "The Magic of the Family Meal," wherein author Nancy Gibbs asserted, "there is something about a shared meal—not some holiday blowout, not once in a while but regularly, reliably—that anchors a family even on nights when the food is fast and the talk cheap and everyone has someplace else they'd rather be. And on those evenings when the mood is right and the family lingers, caught up in an idea or an argument explored in a shared safe place where no one is stupid or shy or ashamed, you get a glimpse of the power of this habit."

And don't let the idea of dinner conjure up any stress of impossible schedules and endless sporting events. Let go of the perfection—just making it happen is what matters.

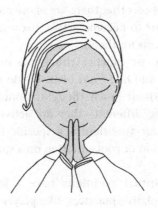

HAVE FAITH

What if you opened yourself to the possibility that there is something greater than us: a spiritual or divine presence in the world that we are all connected to?

Perhaps you already have a strong sense of a spiritual connection at the center of your life, or perhaps it's something quite outside the usual realm of your thinking. Religion can be a touchy subject, but a sense of *faith* in something, some force that we can't quite see but trust is there in a positive, supportive way, can be instrumental in healing and finding balance in our lives.

Neuroscientist Dr. Andrew Newberg observed actual changes in the brain scans of people who had experiences of "being in God's presence." When they look at people who partake in religious and spiritual practices, the research shows that there are many more areas of the brain that start to become active, because it's not just a cognitive process for them.

Every day, we practice rituals: we brush our teeth, eat breakfast, and make our beds. We do them with ease and often without much thought. Contemplative practices aren't too different—they are activities that guide us to direct our attention to a specific focus, often an inward reflection or concentration on a specific sensation or concept.

Many spiritual traditions have a long history of using contemplative practices, like prayer or meditation, to increase compassion, empathy, and attention, as well as quiet the mind. The repetition of prayer, meditation, or chanting, and the consciousness we bring to it, makes it sacred.

Prayer, specifically, may elicit the relaxation response, along with feelings of hope, gratitude, and compassion—all of which have a positive effect on overall well-being. There are several types of prayer, many of which are rooted in the belief that there is a higher power that has some level of influence over our lives. This belief can provide a sense of comfort and support in difficult times and a sense of connection and gratitude in fortunate times.

According to research, healthy centenarians living within Blue Zones usually have a strong connection to faith. The Sardinians and Nicoyans are mostly Catholic. Okinawans in Japan have a blended religion that emphasizes ancestral worship. Centenarians in Loma Linda, California, are Seventh-day Adventists. Ikarians have traditionally been Greek Orthodox. All belong to strong religious communities. The simple act of worship seems to improve our chances of living longer, healthier lives.

It's possible that this is because belonging to a religious or spiritual community fosters larger social networks as well as the adherence to scheduled time during services for self-reflection, prayer, song, and a quiet mind. Most people have a hard time grasping concepts outside of themselves that they can't see or touch, so it appears that gathering together helps to reinforce faith and prayer, meditation, and a sense of belonging.

But let me clarify: religion and faith are not to be confused. It doesn't matter if you identify as Christian, Buddhist, Jewish, Muslim, or Hindu; it appears that people who practice *any* faith have lower rates of cardiovascular disease, depression, stress, and suicide, and their immune systems seem to work better.

In fact, the spiritual practice of recognizing the interconnectedness of all life can also help buffer the pain that comes with difficult experiences, including chronic disease. Researcher Kristin Neff states, "If we can compassionately remind ourselves in moments of falling down that failure is part of the shared human experience, then that moment becomes one of togetherness rather than isolation. When our troubled, painful experiences are framed by the recognition that countless others have undergone similar hardships, the blow is softened."

An exhaustive review that compared spirituality and religiousness to other health interventions found that people with a strong spiritual life often lived longer and had an 18 percent reduction in mortality. Giancarlo Lucchetti, the lead author of the study, calculates that the life-extending benefits of spirituality can be compared to eating a high amount of fruits and vegetables or taking blood pressure medication. Although some researchers have suggested that the extent of spirituality's benefit on health is exaggerated, most researchers agree there is a positive relationship between religious and spiritual practices and better health outcomes. Forgiveness, or letting go of blame and negative feelings after a hurtful incident, is a practice that is reflected by a number of spiritual traditions, including Christianity, Islam, Buddhism, and Judaism.

Researchers at NYU Langone Medical Center have conducted a study of patients who have experienced near-death experiences, and the results are intriguing. Critical care physician Dr. Sam Parnia, the director of resuscitation research, reports that when a person dies, part of what makes us who we are—our soul or consciousness—continues on at least in the early moments of death, when the brain is not expected to be fully functioning.

When I was 25 years old, I was confronted with my own death. I was jogging across the parking lot of my auto mechanic's shop to pick up my car, only to be met by two 120-pound, aggressive Akita attack dogs that had knocked over an employee who was bringing them out of a cage in the back of the building for their nightly shift as guard dogs. I was the first thing they saw when they rounded the corner of the building. I knew immediately they would kill me and that it would be a violent way to die. Once their teeth penetrated the flesh of my leg and arm, I went into shock.

I completely left my physical body in that moment and returned moments later to the sensation of two employees prying open the locked jaws of the two dogs and putting me in the back of a van to rush me to the hospital.

What happened to me that day made me keenly aware that we are not alone in our journey through life. Something bigger than me decided it was not my time to go.

Scientifically, our brains prove that it doesn't matter what we call our God. It's more about what we believe in our hearts. Experiencing the divine actually does change us for the better.

Today, there is a global decline in religion. Younger Americans no longer have the strong ties to organized religion that their parents did. But still, religion and spirituality don't go away easily, or even at all. They have been with us for so long because they seem so rooted in who we are biologically, socially, culturally, and perhaps evolutionarily. At its core, our faith in God is deep-rooted in the expectation of good things to come. It usually shows up one step beyond hope. While much of hope lives in the mind, faith is anchored in the heart.

Faith is not unreachable. My God lives deep inside of me. When we acknowledge what is sacred in all people and all things, we see God as *love* that unites us all. As Fr. Richard Rohr so elegantly expressed in his book *The Universal Christ*, "God loves things by becoming them."

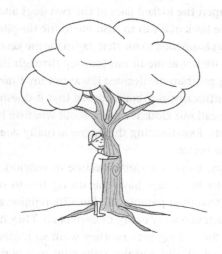

CONNECT
WITH NATURE

A growing body of research shows that simply being present and opening our senses to the sights, sounds, smells, and sensations of the natural world—even for short amounts of time—can decrease our stress levels and improve mood, cognition, focus, and immune system functioning.

"Biophilia" was originally defined in medical dictionaries in the early 1900s as the instinct for self-preservation or the instinctual drive to stay alive. By 1984, Harvard biologist E. O. Wilson expanded the term, proposing biophilia to describe that humans inherently enjoy the diversity of life on earth and that much of our well-being comes from that enjoyment. Wilson's definition of "biophilia" extended to the emotional plane, including matters of mental health and cognitive behavior.

We're all born with an intuitive sense of the healing power of nature: spending time in a forest activates the vagus nerve, which is responsible for inducing calm and regeneration. Spending just one single day in a wooded area can boost the immune system by increasing the number of natural killer cells in the blood by almost 40 percent.

Leisurely forest walks, compared with urban walks, show an over 12 percent decrease in the stress hormone cortisol, a 7 percent decrease in sympathetic nerve activity, a decrease in blood pressure, and a decrease in heart rate. Improvements in immune function have been associated with lower urinary stress hormones while in nature. None of this has been observed during or after comparable trips in the city.

While the reduction in stress is most likely at play in the improvement of immune defenses, we also know the natural chemicals secreted by evergreen trees, collectively known as phytoncides, have also been associated with improvements in the activity of our frontline immune defenders. Research shows that phytoncides in the air correlated to improvements in immune function. The results seemed to be magnified when the forest air trapped moisture.

Geosmin, meaning "earth smell" in Greek, is produced by *Streptomyces*, a genus of the gram-positive bacteria phylum Actinobacteria. Humans are very sensitive to geosmin and can detect it at levels as low as five parts per trillion. Geosmin is one of several molecules that you can smell after it rains. In a 1964 *Nature* article, researchers I. J. Bear and R. G. Thomas analyzed air from rainstorms and found ozone, geosmin, and also aromatic plant oils. The name given to the characteristic odor of rain *after* it rains, especially following a dry spell, is *petrichor*. During dry spells, some plants release the oil, which is absorbed into clay and soil around the plant. The purpose of the oil is to slow seed germination and growth, since it would be unlikely for the seedlings to prosper with insufficient water.

Billions of microorganisms exist in a single tablespoon of soil, including a beneficial strain of bacteria known as Mycobacterium vaccae, or M. vaccae, that can improve cognition and even lower some risk factors of certain brain disorders, such as dementia and Alzheimer's disease. Researchers at The Sage Colleges in New York fed live M. vaccae to mice, then measured their ability to navigate a maze compared to control mice not fed the bacteria. Mice that were fed live M. vaccae navigated the maze twice as fast and with less anxiety. The M. vaccae makes us feel better, and when we spend time outdoors, we breathe it in through the air.

The Japanese version of natural therapy is called *shinrin-yoku*, or forest bathing, which requires patients to walk for extended periods through forested areas while inhaling "woodsy scents" that complement the sylvan atmosphere. Tokyo's Nippon Medical School studied a group of women to investigate the effect of forest bathing on natural killer cells and anti-cancer proteins in the human body. This group spent two to four hours in the woods on two consecutive days and experienced a nearly 50 percent increase in the activity of cancer-fighting white blood cells, and the effect lasted at least seven days after the trip.

While many studies point to the psychological effects we feel in nature, the aromatic substances the plants use to communicate may also be responsible for some of the physiological effects, like lowering your blood pressure. These effects are believed to be linked to terpenes, phytochemicals mainly produced by trees, of which there are more than 40,000 structures reported so far. For example, the smell of cedar oil has been shown to lower blood pressure. But in nature, you have the benefit of breathing in a wide range of potent compounds instead just one isolated oil. To date, many terpenes from essential oils, as well as forest bathing, have been reported to exhibit strong biological activities.

According to Columbia University researchers, other elements found in nature, like negative ions—particles that are plentiful near waterfalls, breaking waves, and river rapids—can also act as natural antidepressants. An *Indoor Air* study found that after breathing negative ions for an hour, subjects' blood lactate levels dropped 33 percent, improving their energy levels.

Of course, nature is not a panacea, but it's an inexpensive and effective tool for dampening the impact of illness and lifting the burden of your everyday stress. A walk in the woods trumps a plant in your office, which trumps a picture of the forest, no matter how soothing. Something deep within us responds to the innate connection to nature, which in my opinion has the potential to tip the balance toward health and resiliency for all of us.

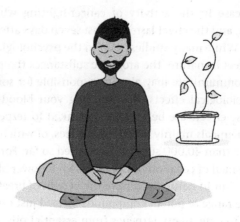

PRESS PAUSE

In a world that that never sleeps, the ability to quiet the mind and the body—including digestion—is essential. You may be surprised to learn that taking an extended pause from eating can improve your health by altering your metabolism and immune function. Perhaps you are familiar with the term "intermittent fasting," the concept of abstaining from food for a set period of time. Time-restricted fasting is one way to burn fat without dieting. Fasting allows you to access fat as a fuel source of energy rather than the steady flow of calories you consume through your diet. It also increases the levels of human growth hormone, which promotes fat loss, muscle growth, health, and longevity.

Biochemist Valter Longo has devoted decades to discovering connections between fasting and longevity. He runs the USC Leonard Davis School of Gerontology's Longevity Institute, which aims to extend healthy lifespans and find ways to prevent and treat aging-related conditions, like cancer and cardiovascular disease. Research indicates that an extended fasting period—ideally a period of 12 hours without food—allows the digestive system the time to rest and restore the integrity of its intestinal walls, or epithelium, as well as allow cellular autophagy (cellular turnover) to occur. This may be especially important to protect us against gut permeability prompted by a poor diet and inflammation that lets bacteria and other toxins enter surrounding tissues.

It turns out that a cycle of fasting and feeding triggers a regenerative process. Intermittent fasting that falls in the range of 12 to 16 hours can also increase insulin sensitivity, reduce inflammation, enhance tissue repair, boost mitochondrial function, rid the body of damaged cells, and increase resilience and longevity. For most people, I recommend starting with an extended fasting period overnight by avoiding food after dinner until your breakfast the following morning. This will allow you to accomplish a 13-hour fast period, which in human observational studies has been associated with reduced risk of breast cancer recurrence in women, reduced risk of elevated HbA1c (glycated hemoglobin, which is associated with glucose in the blood, of which high levels are associated with diabetes), and reduced inflammation.

Fasting is not a new health trend; it has been practiced for centuries in many cultures around the world as a way of maintaining health and youthful vigor. Contrary to popular belief, the goal of intermittent fasting is not to lose weight; it is to give your body a chance to repair itself. I prefer using the term *intermittent silence*, or simply learning to *press pause*, as it removes the notion of deprivation often associated with fasting. When you intentionally pause from consuming any form of stimulation of the senses, you are consciously choosing to abstain with the goal of initiating healing and restoration. You can decide, based on your current circumstances, how long your fasting period should last and consult with your doctor if you have any concerns.

Historically, fasting has coexisted with spiritual practices such as meditation and prayer. This is because the body is in a state of repair, and less attention is being given to the physical form. Buddhism, Hinduism, Judaism, and the Muslim traditions all practice fasting during spiritual events. The *vipassana* practice is a type of silent meditation observed by Buddhists. It is one of the oldest known methods and generally takes place over a 10-day period. Vipassana can be translated as "seeing clearly" or "insight," as in lending clear awareness of exactly what is happening as it happens. It is a state in which the mind is brought to rest, focused only on one goal and not allowed to wander.

The brain is the most complex and powerful organ, and like the gut, it too benefits from rest, not just sleep. Research from UCLA showed that setting aside regular time to disengage, sit in silence, and *mentally* rest improves the "folding" of the cortex and boosts your ability to process information. Even carving out as little as 10 minutes to sit quietly and visualize a peaceful scenery can thicken gray matter in your brain.

In silence, you gain the self-awareness to be in control of your actions rather than letting them control you. The break from external voices puts you in tune with your inner voices and your actions. This self-awareness leads to control, and choosing not to respond to every actionable thought strengthens your willpower. Silence can serve as a doorway to your soul. We live in an age of unprecedented anxiety. Spending all our time trying to anticipate and plan for the future and lamenting the past, we forget to embrace the here and now. We are so concerned with tomorrow that we forget to enjoy today.

Silence and solitude are meant to give us the space to reflect, play catch-up with our thoughts, and nourish our physical and mental well-being. Disengage from the projects at hand, work, and the Internet for a mental break, and take a rest. This will also help you with mental blocks and provide creative clarity.

Combining solitude with a walk in nature can also stimulate the hippocampus region of the brain, resulting in better memory. Evolutionists explain that combining solitude with time in nature sparks our spatial memory, as it did when our ancestors went hunting—remembering where food and predators lay was essential for survival.

Taking a quiet walk without music or conversation can support the brain in achieving uninterrupted focus and helps with memory consolidation. This behavior is really about becoming fully present in your body without relying on the clamor of our modern lifestyle to drown out the voice of your soul. We often desire more clarity to discover what really matters to us—*press pause* to create the space you deserve for self-reflection.

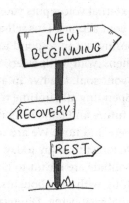

HONOR YOUR
TRANSITIONS

All cultures recognize the need to ritualize major life transitions—changes that have happened or are expected to happen. These changes are often events like births, marriage, or even death, and they tend to fall into categories like beginnings, unions, or endings. But what about healing—the transition out of chronic illness? It's the end of a period of suffering and the beginning of a new phase of health.

But this is a gray (and messy) area between our darkest days and the time we are just starting to see the light at the end the tunnel. How do you honor the space between your time of great struggle and a new beginning? Well, by understanding the role of ritual in your life and marking the point on your journey where you get to hang up your warrior cape and begin focusing on rebuilding your health rather than overcoming disease. Create a ritual, or any symbolic act, that is focused on fulfilling a particular intention that serves to honor your transition.

With so much chronic disease in the world, there are millions of people who spend a good portion of their lives (in some cases several years) coping with illness or fighting disease. But there is no manual that gives you the guidelines to navigate the transition *out* of illness and into a life of optimal health. Most of us don't even know what this transition looks like and how to honor that moment when it arises. Sometimes, it takes someone else to point out that you have survived and your battle is officially over.

For me, it happened during the filming of our documentary film. It was still very difficult for me to talk about my story and my healing journey without crying. I had been asked to recount so much of my journey, including the surgery that left me disabled, the memory of losing the job I loved, and the physical and emotional pain of rehabilitation. At one point, I was asked to put on my body cast, which brought up intense emotions of those early days when my future was so uncertain. One of the producers stopped filming and suggested we take a break. She sat me down, put her hands on my shoulders, and said, "It's over; you did it. You don't have to fight anymore." That was the first time anyone had ever told me that I had won. I beat my chronic disease, and it wasn't ever going to take me back to that dark place. The victory was mine. In that moment, someone was acknowledging that it was time to put my stake in the ground and honor my transition. And it was life-changing. Going forward, that became my ritual—my private ceremony, my mantra—when I hit a crossroads on my journey.

One important, but often neglected, factor in the transition from sickness to health is in how people *perceive* their illness. If you see it as a never-ending journey, you just keep carrying the torch. Of course, depending of your circumstances, transitions will look different for everyone. It's not about assigning a timeline to an illness or a recovery plan but instead about visualizing where you are in the process and identifying different turning points. You can learn to acknowledge when it's time to change direction, begin again, or simply rest.

If you are dealing with a complex illness, it may be helpful to set an intention for your healing. Draw out a plan that includes what your illness looks like to you. An article published in January 2018 in the journal *Health Psychology Review* explored how well drawings of an illness correspond to how patients think of their illness, how they'll cope, and ultimately how likely they are to get healthy again. The idea that drawing an illness can offer insights into our state of mind and health outcomes is fascinating. In the 101 research papers that the researchers reviewed, they found surprising correlations between different aspects of patients' drawings and their health outcomes. For example, heart-attack patients who drew hearts with larger areas of damage had larger damage, took longer to return to work, and believed that they had less control and that their recovery would take longer.

A similar effect was seen in patients with traumatic brain injury. When they drew their brains, a greater number of damaged areas in the drawing was associated with greater consequences from their condition, a worse quality of life, more symptoms, a longer recovery time, and other variables.

Why does this matter? We often spend incredible amounts of time and energy fighting what is really happening. It can be difficult to see what's happening when we are living it every day—physically and emotionally. For change to occur, you must admit what is true and accept it. When you let go of the resistance, the pain loosens its grip, and change can occur.

Transitions signify moving toward something new and even unfamiliar. The research on drawings demonstrates that those exercises could provide insights into a wide variety of perceptions and sensations when it comes to illnesses. It also made me think about the aspects of change that accompany healing, including the loss of what was and the unknown of what lies ahead. These changes can make the healing experience even more difficult. Even when the change is a sought-after improvement, it's not uncommon to feel uncertain as we shift to find our sense of wholeness again. You will realize the wholeness is never really lost; you just lost touch with it.

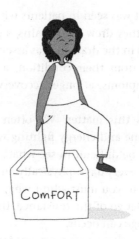

COMFORT

TAKE ACTION

Knowledge is power, but execution leads to *results*. If you want to heal, you must take action. When you change your patterns, you gain control of your biology. In Part I, I talked about *wisdom* and how to embody self-knowledge as the foundation of regenerating and optimizing your health. This behavior puts that belief into motion.

Knowledge becomes wisdom through personal experience, which involves action. I used to consume information like some people devour a bag of potato chips—I couldn't stop. To some extent, I still find myself overconsuming health-related books, research, podcasts, seminars, and educational programs without factoring the time and effort required to apply most of it to my life or even my clinical practice.

I noticed the same behavior in my clients. They had so much knowledge of their specialized diets; massive amounts of diagnostic data in the form of lab tests, reports, and self-assessments; plus information from countless online programs and seminars they had participated in. They understood the latest trends and followed all the advice from the health gurus. And yet they were not any further along in their understanding of how to achieve wellness nor able to effectively move past their illness. In some cases, they were worse off. They, as I did at one time, felt even more confused about what the root problem was before they had started searching for answers. I began to question whether knowing too much was a deficit rather than a blessing. Does accumulating excess knowledge about our illness or healing hinder our ability to see clearly?

I think it was best articulated by business entrepreneur Jim Kwik when he shared this message with his social media audience: "Knowledge is not power, it is potential power. Execution is understanding." When you take action, you apply your knowledge, and you gain wisdom and understanding of the information. You begin to understand what things apply to you and, perhaps more important, what things don't. You must become obsessed with asking yourself the following question: "How will I use this information in *my* life?" Then do it. Learn. Apply. Repeat.

If you struggle with intellectual curiosity that keeps you gathering more information, set parameters for what you need to know now. If the information you have now provides enough answers to move you forward, take the first step. This approach will continue to give you clarity on how to make progress while avoiding overwhelm.

Of course, we all want to be moving toward vibrant health, but everyone will inevitably get sick or have setbacks from time to time. When you do get sick or hit a bump in the road, how will you recover? What will this process of restoring health look like? Being prepared with a plan *before* the worst happens is critical to your success in ending the cycle of chronic disease. Building a wellness team puts you in the driver's seat before acute illness strikes, and it keeps you on the path to wellness.

We have become adept at identifying acute issues like a fever because we recognize what our normal body temperature should be. However, the sudden onset of symptoms may be indicative of the body being out of balance and in need of restoration. The process of restoration is more complex, and the type of imbalances can be challenging for us to identify on our own, particularly if we are struggling with chronic disease or raising a sick child. The benefit of building a wellness team to support you—in sickness *and* in health—can offset these challenges. You might include some combination of practitioners, like a chiropractor, acupuncturist, nutritionist, massage therapist, health coach, midwife, naturopathic physician, or nurse practitioner.

We need to rethink what health means from birth to death and how we can actively maintain it throughout our life. Resilient health begins at home with quality food, proper sleep, a nontoxic environment, and natural remedies for strengthening immune health. But it also means being exposed to a wide range of healing disciplines that honor the whole person. It does not reject the need for allopathic medicine, but instead considers your *entire* picture of health, and emphasizes self-care and community as the foundation so that you can avoid impulsive choices when you do fall ill.

Find practitioners and techniques that work *with* you, not against your efforts. Most people don't realize that chiropractic adjustments allow our entire body to begin the process of restoration and have even been shown to alter the sensory processing system in the prefrontal cortex of the brain. When left unchecked, physical and emotional stress accumulates in our body and impacts our nervous system.

Curating a conscious support team will contribute to your ability to allow healing to take place in the body's necessary time frame. You will also learn that not every healthcare provider is meant to help everyone. Fear can destroy even the most effective medicine, while compassionate care and faith in a plan can move mountains. You have to engage in the medicine that is right for you. Working with practitioners that are aligned with you will make all the difference in your health outcomes.

Our healthcare system that treats and manages chronic disease with drugs and surgery is not broken. It was built to shape our culture a certain way, to shape our views about health in a way that keeps certain people— the pharmaceutical industry—in a dominant position. It was built for profit and political power. It's incumbent upon each of us to take action in our own lives—to opt out of a dysfunctional system that only thrives if we remain ignorant. Even the majority of doctors and nurses caring for chronically ill patients share this frustration.

To live your best life, you can't just admire others for being their best or retain the knowledge of what needs to happen. One requirement to apply to all things in life, whether it's healing, achieving professional success, or mastering your personal goals, is essentially the same for all individuals: take action. Create that momentum by taking the first step, and then keep going. Results will follow.

Part III

BACTERIA

Bacteria have learned to live in every part of the earth, from the hottest to the coldest, no matter how dangerous, so they have no problem living inside or on us! Many of the bacteria we come into contact with every day are actually helpful.

Bacteria get a lot of bad press, but they don't deserve it all—there are lots of bacteria that play an important role for all living things on earth. In ecological settings, different species are always interacting. It's actually all about relationships. If you acknowledge that you yourself are an ecosystem, you can begin to appreciate the relationships that develop when organisms share a common space—including your body. Some experts believe we should be seen as *holobionts* (ecological units comprising many different species), a term that reflects the intimate, codependent relationship humans have with microbes.

Humans have an invisible coating of microorganisms—a complex mix of bacteria, viruses, archaea, and fungi—that live in communities. There are three common relationships in which humans and bacteria coexist symbiotically: *commensalism*, *mutualism*, and *parasitism*. Commensalism is a relationship that is beneficial to the bacteria but does not help or harm us. Most commensal bacteria reside on epithelial surfaces, like the skin and respiratory tract, that come in contact with the external environment, as well as in the gastrointestinal tract. Commensal bacteria acquire nutrients and a place to live and grow from their hosts. In some instances, commensal bacteria may become pathogenic and cause disease, or they may provide a benefit for the host.

In a mutualistic relationship, both the bacteria and we benefit, as the name implies. There are several kinds of mutualistic bacteria that live on the skin or inside the mouth, nose, throat, or intestines. In exchange for a place to live, these bacteria keep harmful microbes from taking up residence. Bacteria in the digestive system also assist in nutrient metabolism, vitamin production, and waste processing, as well as aiding in the immune response to pathogenic bacteria.

A parasitic relationship is one in which the bacteria benefit while we, the hosts, may be harmed. Pathogenic parasites, which can cause disease, do so by resisting our defenses and growing at our expense. These bacteria produce toxic by-products or substances called endotoxins or exotoxins, which are responsible for many of the symptoms we experience with an illness. Parasitic bacteria are responsible for a number of diseases, including meningitis, pneumonia, tuberculosis, and several types of foodborne illness.

But all things considered, bacteria are more helpful than harmful. We have exploited bacteria for a wide variety of beneficial uses—making cheese and butter, decomposing waste in sewage plants, and developing lifesaving antibiotics. The more scientists learn about microorganisms and what they are doing, the more we realize they are a vital part of what it means to be a fully functioning human. Normal flora consists of communities of bacteria that function as microbial ecosystems and perform many physiological, nutritional, and protective functions in the human body, depending on their location.

Many different bacteria live inside the gut, and we are lucky to have them on board. Bacteria in our gut make lots of copies of themselves. In fact, if they do a good enough job replicating themselves, there should be little room for bad bacteria to take up residence! The good bacteria don't grow too big because there is only a certain amount of resources, the things like food, space, and so on, that they need to grow. When they reach the limit of the resources, they are in equilibrium with your gut. Dysbiosis, on the other hand, is an imbalance in which the good bacteria are unhappy because an unhealthy invader has overcrowded them and their living arrangements are now compromised.

A particular type of good bacteria that lives in the gut is called *Bifidobacterium*. The word *bifido* just means "split into two"—forming its shape like a *Y* with two ears called "lobes"—and *bacterium* just means a single bacteria! Members of the genus *Bifidobacterium* were among the first microbes to colonize the human gastrointestinal tract and are believed to bestow positive health benefits on us.

Bacteria come in various shapes and sizes and thrive in the body, on the skin, and on objects we use every day. Everything living in one ecology is called its *flora* or *microbiota*. The *microbiome* is the broader term, which encompasses both the microbiota as well as their genetic elements—in other words, the organisms and their DNA and how they interact with the host (that is to say, you). The microbiome also includes the metabolic by-products that these organisms produce.

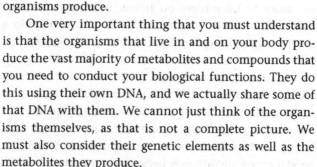

One very important thing that you must understand is that the organisms that live in and on your body produce the vast majority of metabolites and compounds that you need to conduct your biological functions. They do this using their own DNA, and we actually share some of that DNA with them. We cannot just think of the organisms themselves, as that is not a complete picture. We must also consider their genetic elements as well as the metabolites they produce.

To add some context to this subject, the latest estimate, according to the Human Genome Project, shows that human DNA has about 19,000 genes. This finding reveals a shocking truth: that we have less information in our DNA than we previously thought. Bacteria, on the other hand, were found to have a staggering 3.5 million genes.

With at least 150 to 200 times more microbial genetic information in your body than human genetic information, it's clear that you use this microbial DNA in order to function as a human being—that is, to breathe, walk, metabolize food, fight disease, etc. In short, *without our bacteria, we couldn't function*.

Bacteria have a lot to teach us when it comes to combating chronic disease and maintaining health, as some are capable of living in the most extreme environments. Bacteria have also demonstrated that they are able to survive without us. We, on the other hand, could not live without them. We are just beginning to learn the depth of their true nature and the complexity of our relationship with them. But what we know for certain is that we have a lot to learn from them.

Our resiliency hinges on our willingness to learn from them and to acknowledge that they bring far more to our lives than the risk of disease. I cannot overstate the impact or influence that your bacteria have on your daily life. In fact, very few microbes are even harmful—less than one percent of bacteria that invade our body actually makes us ill. The best way to control the few microbes that could be dangerous to human health is to allow the good bacteria that live in, on, and around us to flourish.

We know that when people are suffering from severe allergies, food intolerances, or autoimmune diseases, the microbiome is playing a role. Even when the digestive system is not involved and allergies are not at play, the microbiome is involved in conditions like anxiety or even depression. As much as nutrition and functional medicine are advancing awareness of the microbiome's role in most chronic illnesses, the challenge, of course, is figuring out how to properly identify the dysfunction of the microbiome and how to go about treating it.

Most of the time, a well-meaning practitioner will start with prescribing antimicrobials in an attempt to clean things up, then maybe follow that with various probiotics and prebiotics, and perhaps some supportive supplements like aloe or licorice root to repair and restore overall gut health. This may or may not lead to some improvement for a short period. Unfortunately, this approach fails to address the fundamental issues that occur within the microbiome, or what I call the core foundation of building your inner ecology: the quality and diversity of our microbial allies.

Within the gut you have a mucosal layer, where the majority of your beneficial bacteria reside. They conduct many of their functions there, including receiving information from immune cells, which sit below in the mucin layer. Of course, I am oversimplifying the symphony that happens as the immune cells cross-talk with the microbiome. But in essence, the bacteria are training the immune system by sampling what you are exposed to in order to decide what is friend or foe. These layers are also intentionally separated and defined regions of the gut. When these layers begin to break down, chronic disease begins to set in. Low diversity and low quality, which we'll learn more about in this section, leads to disruption of the mucosal layer and higher risk for infections, chronic inflammation, food intolerances, and environmental sensitivities.

While our bacteria do the important work of keeping pathogens in check, as well as helping us digest the fiber in our food and producing vitamins for us, they also train the immune system in how to respond when we are in danger. There are two genomes—ours and our bacteria's—in cahoots, sending messages back and forth to one another, to sustain our bodies.

In this section, we'll explore some of the key lessons bacteria can teach us in our effort to regenerate health and end the vicious cycle of chronic illness once and for all.

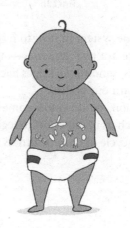

SETTING THE STAGE: FIRST 1,000 DAYS

Microbial colonization of the intestines begins during infancy and plays an instrumental role in the development of the immune system. Our ability to maintain immune tolerance is really a matter of how the immune system is trained in the first thousand days of life—and beyond. The trainer is the *microbiome*.

During pregnancy, a mother begins the inoculation of her baby's microbiome by transferring microbes from her mouth to the placenta. Researchers speculate that they come from the mother's blood, which contains small amounts of mouth bacteria—likely transferred there during normal teeth brushing. It appears the mouth-to-womb connection goes both ways; pregnancy may induce changes in the oral microbiome of the mother. Studies on placental microbes are still being worked out, but perhaps this gives us insight into how microbes are priming us for our exposure to the external world long before our grand entrance.

The birth canal is also part of the inoculation process, as the infant inherits some helpful bacteria from the vaginal microbiome, and this microbiome starts to shift as pregnancy progresses. The vast majority of bacteria within the vaginal tract of a nonpregnant woman are *Lactobacillus crispatus*. The prevalence of this species is actually a good indication of a healthy vaginal microbiome. What happens by the second trimester of pregnancy is that another species—*Lactobacillus johnsonii* (*L. johnsonii*)—becomes the boss. The function of *L. johnsonii* is to help the baby digest and metabolize colostrum and breast milk from the mother. Because babies do not produce enzymes in the early days of life, the microbiome plays a *critical* role in the digestive process.

Studies have also shown that babies born vaginally have higher levels of *Bifidobacteria*, which are species that help to stimulate the immune system and mature the gut lining. In contrast, babies born via caesarean section lack this type of beneficial bacteria and as a result miss this early phase of immune stimulation. The link between these colonizing bacteria and the immune system— together with other factors—could explain why caesarean section babies are statistically five times more likely to develop allergies, have triple the risk of developing ADHD, double the risk of autism, an 80 percent increase in the risk of celiac disease, and a 50 percent increase in the risk of becoming obese as an adult.

In the early days of life, the baby's microbiome will match that of its mother's. Over the next few months, the baby's microbiome will shift to match the mother's skin microbiome, then shift to reflect other members of the family. Early skin-to-skin contact, also called kangaroo care, has been shown to ease babies into the work of regulating their body temperature and heart rate, as well as increasing their breastfeeding success. It also strengthens the immune system, particularly for babies that are born prematurely or via C-section and that may be more vulnerable to allergies and infections.

As the environment changes, the microbes will shift accordingly. The microbiome will also shift in accordance to the baby's behaviors. This is referred to as the *microbiome succession*. Breastfeeding, for example, will provide up to 800 different species of microbes via the breast milk as well as up to 200 different prebiotic oligosaccharides. The sole purpose of the oligosaccharides in the breast milk is strictly to feed the microbiome, which will improve the function of the baby's immune system.

Recent studies have begun to define critical periods during early development in which disruption of our microbiome can lead to persistent and in some cases *irreversible* defects, including the development of diseases later in life such as inflammatory bowel disease, allergies, and asthma.

A 2015 study published in *Pediatrics* linked childhood antibiotic use and microbiome disturbance to autoimmune conditions, including an increased risk of developing juvenile idiopathic arthritis (JIA) with any antibiotic exposure—even after factoring out the infections the children were being treated for. In addition, antibiotic-treated upper respiratory tract infections were more strongly associated with JIA than untreated upper respiratory tract infections. The more antibiotics given, the higher the risk of disease.

This is important because one quarter of the antibiotic prescriptions for children—and approximately half of those prescriptions for acute respiratory infection—may be unnecessary.

Although you certainly can't go back and change how you were born or how you were fed as an infant, there's power in knowing what we can do to support a newborn's developing microbiome for future generations. We can also counteract any negative effects from a compromised microbiome by implementing the lifestyle *behaviors* discussed in this book that increase the diversity of your gut microbes and in turn reduce your risk of developing chronic diseases as an adult.

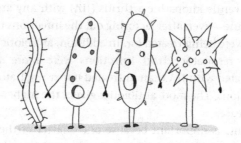

BIODIVERSITY IS KEY

Bacterial biodiversity paves the way for good health and long-term resiliency. Low diversity of bacterial strains equals a higher risk for chronic illness, including a decrease in longevity and higher mortality. Biodiversity—a term we often hear in agriculture but not gut health—refers to the richness of your microbiome: the total number of bacterial species in our gut as well as the number of individual bacteria from each of those bacteria species present.

Our gut microbiome is a vast community of trillions of bacteria (and fungi) that inhabit every fold of the intestinal tract and have a major influence on our body weight, mood, appetite, and propensity to illness. Dysbiosis, or low levels of good bacteria, has been linked to higher risks for infections, chronic inflammation, and food intolerances. The richer and more diverse the community of gut microbes are, the lower the risk of disease and allergies. This has been shown in human studies comparing bacteria of people with and without specific diseases like diabetes, obesity, allergies, colitis, and arthritis. An extended benefit of having a rich bacterial community thriving within us is their ability to help protect us from pathogens, common germs, and even environmental chemicals.

When it comes to detoxification, we often think of many plant-based foods and supplementation to support our natural cleansing processes and increase our capacity to handle stress, but our gut bacteria are also working on our behalf to protect us from environmental toxins on a daily basis. Microbes can also offer protection against our exposure to heavy metals, like lead, cadmium, mercury, and the metalloid arsenic, that can cause symptoms of nausea, heart problems, headaches, central nervous system dysfunction, and other chronic illnesses. The bacteria strain *Lactobacillus rhamnosus* GR~1 has been shown to block absorption of arsenic and mercury. *Lactobacillus* has also been shown to increase the amounts of heavy metals expelled in stool, meaning it too has the ability to mitigate their presence in the body.

In addition to heavy metals, some bacteria can also protect us from exposure to potentially damaging plastics. Bisphenol A, or BPA, is one such example that has been linked to potential effects on the brain, behavior, and prostate glands in fetuses, infants, and young children.

While, thankfully, many products that once contained high levels of BPA have been repackaged, it's still possible to be exposed to this harmful chemical through food and water. The good news is that certain strains of bacteria actually digest carcinogens like BPA. *Lactobacillus casei* and *Bifidobacterium breve* were found to bind to BPA, offsetting the amount that would otherwise wind up in our bloodstream.

Many diseases are accompanied by dramatic changes in the makeup of our inner ecosystems, driving the diversity of bacteria down and compressing quality. The association between reduced diversity and disease indicates that species-rich gut ecosystems are more resilient against environmental influences. Compared to healthy controls, lower bacterial diversity has been observed repeatedly in people with inflammatory bowel disease, psoriatic arthritis, diabetes (type 1 and type 2), atopic eczema, obesity, celiac disease, and arterial stiffness.

New microbes may simply take up residence in our bodies when disease alters the landscape; clinically, we call this an "opportunistic" shift in terrain. In other cases, however, the microbes may help give rise to the disease. It's hard to say what happens first, but diversity seems to be a generally good indicator of a "healthy gut."

What might surprise you is that only a tiny proportion of supplements have been shown to be beneficial in increasing the diversity of our microbiome. The lasting results continue to point to eating a diverse range of real food to get all of the nutrients and at the same time feed our microbes, which in turn expands our bacterial diversity. We also swallow around a million microbes in every gram of food we eat. Microbes are everywhere.

The Hadza people of Tanzania have a gut microbiome diversity that is one of the richest on the planet and about 40 percent higher than the average American's. The Hadza eat around 600 species of plants and animals in a year, along with huge seasonal variation. They have virtually none of the common Western diseases, such as allergies, heart disease, cancer, and obesity. In contrast, we eat fewer than 50 species of plants and animals in our diet, and we are facing an epidemic of chronic illness and obesity.

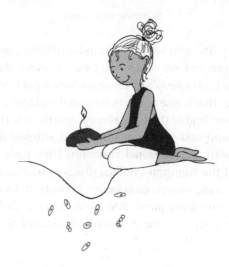

RECONNECT

The *hygiene hypothesis* of stress-related diseases states that because we spend less time in nature and overuse anti-bacterial soaps and other germ-killing aids, our bodies no longer reap the benefits of microbes, which have helped humans survive and thrive for thousands of years. If we listen closely, nature is trying to tell us *we belong together*.

We humans coexist with literally trillions of bacteria, archaea, yeast, mold, other fungi, bacteriophages, viruses, and parasites. Our immune system must be able to tolerate thousands of harmless species while maintaining its ability to attack dangerous pathogens. Scientists are finding that the microbiome *itself,* and the microbes found in nature, guide the immune system to the proper balance.

Despite our inborn appreciation for nature, as a culture, we are still spending too much of our precious time indoors—bathed in artificial light and breathing recycled air. According to the National Academies of Sciences, Engineering, and Medicine, humans spend roughly 90 percent of each day indoors in environments built from man-made materials such as concrete, glass, and plastic. Within these built environments, there does exist a vast number of diverse species of microbes—in the air, the water, and the heating, ventilation, and air-conditioning systems. However, there have been few systematic efforts to collect and describe the microbes living in the constructed environments in which we spend most of our time, and the relative benefit provided by indoor species versus those found in nature are still unclear. Traditionally, the study of indoor microbes has focused on known pathogens or on microbes that can damage a structure—things like black mold on the walls, bacteria linked to respiratory infections, or airborne pathogens. Researchers have focused on the most virulent agents associated with widespread outbreaks or allergic reactions.

What we do know is that reducing our time in nature, where microbes are abundant, coupled with increased time indoors, where the environment is more stagnant, is not reducing chronic disease. With time spent indoors, we have also increased our exposure to technology that our microbes may be sensitive to, and that appears to be a double whammy.

A study compared the growth rate of *Escherichia coli* (*E. Coli*) and *Listeria monocytogenes*—potential pathogens—under conditions of exposure to radio frequencies similar to those emitted by mobile devices or Wi-Fi. They both showed significantly faster growth after radiation exposure, and within six hours of radiation exposure, the *E. coli* became more resistant to antibiotics. *E. coli* is considered a beneficial strain of bacteria in the gut under healthy conditions, but it can also be highly pathogenic, and overgrowth has been implicated in inflammatory bowel diseases such as Crohn's, ulcerative colitis, and irritable bowel syndrome, and is also associated with colorectal cancer.

There are also benefical species commonly found in our intestines that appear to be vulnerable to the detrimental effects of radiation: *Lactobacillus plantarum*, well known for its benefits in healing the intestinal barrier; and *Lactobacillus rhamnosus*, which has a solid track record in improving allergies, gastrointestinal dysfunction, and immunity. Our bacteria help us digest foods, fight off pathogenic infections, regulate our immune function, and properly eliminate waste. To perform these duties, the populations of different types of beneficial bacteria need to be maintained and in proper balance.

It is now clear that maintaining a healthy microbiome is of chief importance in maintaining our health. It seems wise to offset our time spent indoors exposed to technology by reconnecting with a diverse bacterial ecology—Mother Nature. The strategy of reconnecting with our ancient microbial friends and preserving any protective gut bacteria we already have on board to promote optimal health and wellness is one worth considering. Without these microbial allies, our bodies fall prey to the negative effects of stress and chronic inflammation, and this adversely affects our body's ability to prevent disease.

Spending time in nature—city parks, gardens, farms, and uninhabited woods alike—increases our exposure to a diverse microbial community. Get outside and breathe the fresh air as often as you can. After all, longtime nature lovers swear that spending time among plants is therapeutic.

Now we know why.

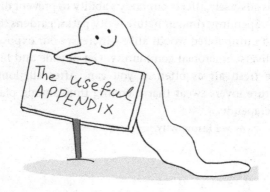

EVERYTHING HAS A PURPOSE

Most of us still have a special little vestigial organ that, per Charles Darwin, once served a necessary function that time has rendered either diminished or nonexistent: the appendix. A research team at Duke University that has traced the appendix back through nearly 80 million years of evolutionary history says the appendix just might do something for the human body besides getting infected.

The appendix is a narrow tube attached to the upper part of the large intestine. Far from its functionless reputation, it is packed full of specialized immune cells called lymphocytes. Once thought to assist primates in digesting leaves, the appendix reveals its true purpose through its contents. It seems to be a depository for a community of beneficial microbial inhabitants.

Researchers have examined tissue from healthy human appendices and discovered biofilms in their lining. We now believe that our good bacteria may actually move out of the intestines and into the appendix so the immune system does not attack them while trying to get rid of an infection. The bacteria residing temporarily in the appendix can be used to repopulate the colon after the infection has passed. In a way, the appendix serves as a safe haven for microbes when the digestive system is out of whack. It seems to safeguard these bacteria against being found by the white blood cells.

We can also think of the appendix as a type of insurance policy against an unexpected bout of food poisoning or a round of antibiotics following a gastrointestinal infection. Inside the appendix, these microbes form this protective biofilm to support one another while excluding bacteria that might cause harm. In our time of need, they repopulate the gut with healthy bacteria, though surgical removal of the appendix does not appear to cause any observable health problems.

Researchers also suggest that the appendix sheds biofilm of mutualistic resident microbes on a regular basis. We know that the gut epithelial tissue has high turnover, that it is constantly shedding and repairing. Evidence suggests the appendix inoculates other sections of the gastrointestinal tract with its biofilms. The appendix is believed to be part of the gut-associated lymphoid tissue (GALT) and playing an immunological role much like that of the tonsils and adenoids (also once considered to be vestigial).

The tonsils are purported to be the body's first line of defense against inhaled or ingested pathogens, but they, like the appendix, have a tendency to join the opposing force and get infected and inflamed. This has led many to question if the tonsils ever served a specific function in the body that outweighed the need to have them removed, as so many do once they have been bothered by repeated infections.

Surprisingly, as part of the lymphatic system, the tonsils play an important role in educating the immune system. Though small, concealed, and seemingly insignificant, tonsils have several meaninful functions when it comes to our well-being. We can first think of them as goalies for the throat, where they prevent foreign objects from slipping into the lungs, filter bacteria and viruses from our environment, and produce white blood cells and antibodies in our defense against invaders. Tonsils also sample bacteria and viruses entering the body through the mouth or nose to educate the rest of the immune system and flush them using lymph, a clear and colorless fluid that runs throughout the body. Some have also linked the tonsils to the glymphatic system in the brain.

So much of the focus on the tonsils up to this point has been around strep throat, and for good reason. Each year, strep throat sickens some 600 million people across the globe. Bacteria called group A *Streptococcus* are to blame, causing symptoms of sore throat, fever, and more. Kids who get the disease are at risk of heart problems and *rheumatic fever*, a noninfectious but very serious disease. For parents, recurring strep infections in children are scary. They are also a problem that has puzzled scientists.

Now a study of kids' tonsils suggests that some kids have a faulty immune response to strep bacteria. Others are misdiagnosed with the disease when strep germs hide out in their tonsils. In this study, researchers at the La Jolla Institute for Immunology in Southern California examined tonsils from kids 5 to 18 years old. Some had had their tonsils taken out because of frequent strep throat. Others had had theirs removed to fix breathing problems caused by large tonsils. The team looked at pieces of the tonsils under a microscope and noticed that kids with recurring strep had smaller immune structures called *germinal centers*. And these centers made fewer immune cells known as T cells. T cells help other immune cells known as B cells make infection-fighting antibodies. Kids with recurring strep had fewer antibodies that respond to a protein in group A strep that helps the microbe mess with the immune system and may leave kids more prone to future infections.

What's important about this research is that we may need to rethink our relationship to bacteria, how our organs work, what their true purpose is, and what role we play in staying well *before* we remove any part of the body. Bacteria are often falsely blamed for illness, when in reality, it's more complicated than that. In fact, in many cases, strep bacteria now live harmlessly in people's tonsils due to some earlier infection. In such cases, a sore throat due to a virus might now be mistaken as strep throat. Tests can turn up signs that the body chronically hosts the group A strep germ, which infectious disease experts estimate happens in 20 percent of school-aged kids.

Of course, in some cases when infection leads to inflammation that cannot be resolved, getting a tonsillectomy or an appendectomy does lead to great improvements in our health. However, these two seemingly passive organs offer a great lesson about how our bodies are working in concert with our microbes as partners in our health.

It seems that holding on to the appendix and the tonsils into adulthood, whenever possible, may bring a number of health benefits, including protection from infections, autoimmune disorders, blood cancer, heart attacks, and immune dysfunction. More importantly, these organs remind us that everything has a purpose and that even the smallest consistent gestures—like shedding biofilms of beneficial microbes—can have a huge impact on our long-term health and defense against chronic disease!

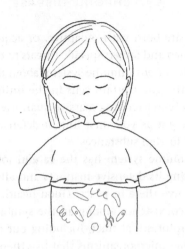

IMMUNITY

Many chronic illnesses that plague us, including asthma, allergy, and inflammatory bowel syndrome, share the common thread of a dysregulated immune system. Immune dysregulation occurs when the immune system remains stuck in an inflammatory response rather than shifting into an adaptive phase; when this occurs, it leaves the body prone to chronic disease and for many, autoimmune diseases. Some clarity about the immune system might be helpful, but don't worry nothing too heavy; you won't need a trowel to get through the weeds of immune system jargon.

The immune can be broadly sorted into two categories: innate and adaptive immunity. Innate, as the name suggests, refers to the functional parts of the immune system we are born with. Adaptive, or acquired, immunity is learned and targets specific threats to the body. The vast majority of our immune system (about 80 percent) is located in the gut. Certain cells in the lining of the gut spend their lives excreting massive quantities of antibodies into the gut as your first line of defense against the invasion of foreign substances.

The immune system has the careful job in the gut of suppressing its defensive instincts and allowing many bacteria to live there in peace. Good health depends on a peaceful coexistence among all the symbiotic bacteria in the gastrointestinal tract, including our cells, tissues, and the other microorganisms that live there as well. At the same time, it must recognize dangerous intruders. The immune system is designed to control microbes but, in essence, the microbes themselves also control immunity.

Our microbes are in constant communication with the immune system on every surface of our bodies and are important for training the immune system throughout life. Our bacteria educate and influence our body's response by serving as a signaling hub that integrates environmental inputs, such as diet, with genetic and immune signals to affect our metabolism and overall response to infection. Strange as it may sound, our microbes may be getting secret messages from some unexpected locations.

Noam Cohen, M.D., Ph.D., head and neck surgeon at the Philadelphia VA hospital, was curious why a small number of his sinus patients never got better after surgery. Were they susceptible to infection in some way that most of the patients, who recovered completely, were not?

It turns out the nose is lined with bitter and sweet taste receptors that may have less to do with helping us taste or smell dinner and more to do with our ability to fight off respiratory infections.

Cohen and his colleagues at University of Pennsylvania, tested samples from the noses of his patients and found that one of the bitter taste receptors in upper airway acts as a type of "security guard" by detecting molecules that a certain class of bacteria secrete.

"Supertasters" are the champions of gastronomy, able to detect even the slightest differences in bitter flavor that most of us miss. About 25 percent of people are supertasters, another 25 percent can barely detect bitterness, and the rest of us fall somewhere in between. When the supertasters' receptors were exposed to the by-product of *Pseudomonas aeruginosa*, a bacterium that is commonly linked to sinus infections, they did two things to help them fend off the bacteria: They activated the tiny hairs in their nose, called cilia, that sweep germs out, and they increased production of nitric oxide, which kills bacteria. People who lacked the genes to taste bitterness did not respond at all.

Cohen's research demonstrates that these receptors are there to detect and fight off pathogens. One implication of their finding is that excess mucosal sugar might prevent this critical immune response from occurring— and protecting the nose. Cohen, for example, discovered that his sinusitis patients have higher levels of sugar in the mucus linings of their noses, making them prone to sinus infections. Other researchers have also confirmed that people prone to sinusitis, as well as diabetics, have on average three to four times the normal amount of sugar in their mucus. Perhaps even more interesting from this perspective, is that our immune and taste systems utilize some of the same chemosensory receptors.

But it turns out that taste receptors for bitterness aren't just in our noses or on our tongues (as you would suspect). Taste receptors have been found in tissue across the human body, including the gastrointestinal tract, bladder, brain, and airway. These extraoral taste receptors appear to be important in modulating the innate immune response through detection of pathogens.

In our lungs, these receptors help control mucus and the production of airflow. Researchers at the University of Maryland School of Medicine in Baltimore tested a few standard bitter substances known to activate these receptors in the lungs and it turns out that the bitter compounds opened the airway more profoundly than any known drug used for treatment of asthma or chronic obstructive pulmonary disease (COPD).

Graduate student Kathryn Winglee, also made a fascinating discovery in the lab of William Bishai of the Johns Hopkins Center for Tuberculosis Research Laboratory. In her study on the role of the gut microbiome in tuberculosis, Winglee infected five mice with TB and then collected stool samples once a month until the mice died and analyzed the genetic material they contained. She found that the TB infection in the lung changed the bacterial communities in the gut significantly. Winglee and her colleagues think that the immune system is sending a signal about infections from lung to gut, which appears to respond by killing off certain microbial species. The next step is to determine why.

Given the microbiota's role in setting the systemic immune tone, scientists are now investigating the role of the commensal microbiota in chronic and autoimmune disease. Since microbes can provide protection against some inflammatory disorders and regulate how much inflammation occurs in the body, it would be wise for us to do whatever we can to protect our microbial partners and acknowledge their role in modulating immune response, including the regulation of innate and adaptive immunity.

We know that our gastrointestinal tract is in direct contact with the outside world with what we eat. This direct interaction between the bacteria in our gut and what we eat is central to our health. From there, it's an easy next step to understand that improving the factors of our environment—that is, choosing high quality food and lifestyle choices—will strengthen the immune system.

This insight on taste receptors suggests that our immunity is contingent on a much more sophisticated dialogue happening inside our body in response to external input. Perhaps, our greatest role is to enhance this complex microbial/cellular conversation rather than bog it down with unnecessary interference.

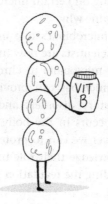

BUILT-IN APOTHECARY

There is no scientific proof that getting our nutrients straight from a pill delivers on the promise to improve our health. Instead, when we eat healthy food, we are investing in a source of nutrition for our microbes and creating a built-in apothecary, if you will. Our gut bacteria actually produce many important nutrients, which makes supporting vitamin-producing gut bacteria a long-term investment that is fueled by the quality of food we consume on a daily basis.

When we are born, *Bifido* species predominate. Over time, *Lacto* species start to take over. Both *Bifidobacterium bifidum* and *Bifidobacterium longum* produce folate, a B vitamin that promotes cell growth, supports the metabolism of proteins, and is critical during pregnancy for normal development and growth of the fetus. Some lactobacilli produce folate as well, and this species is abundant in fermented foods; however, it's unclear if its function would differ from the folate produced by bacteria in the colon, since dietary folate would be absorbed within the small intestine. There may be an important physiological reason that, unlike nutrients found in supplements and foods that are absorbed in the small intestine, nutrients produced by bacteria are absorbed within the large intestine. This may suggest the need to have nutrients in both places for different reasons.

Our gut bacteria produce important vitamins, like B12 and K, and without them we can suffer the consequences of depression, anxiety, and even dementia. The bacteria in the gut secrete and respond to neurotransmitters, including dopamine, serotonin, and GABA, all of which have antidepressant properties in the brain. It's likely that this is one of the primary ways gut bacteria influence our mood.

Although the brain uses neurotransmitters to send messages, it doesn't want a lot of background noise to disturb its delicate signals, which is one of the primary reasons why there's a blood-brain barrier. This complex structure protects our precious brains from all that surrounds them. The blood-brain barrier blocks most neurotransmitters from the gut and the rest of the body. For the same reason, there is also a barrier between the blood and the gut-brain. Still, research does show that these neurotransmitters do have an impact on the brain, and usually the vagus nerve is involved. The bacteria seem to do a good job of turning out quite a bit of neurotransmitter production.

Nurturing specific microbial species can help us set up internal defenses against chronic symptoms as well. *Lactobacillus reuteri*, for example, can dampen pain and calm overly anxious bowels by slowing down peristalsis. It does so by sending the signal to the brain via the vagus nerve that everything is okay in the gut.

There is also growing evidence to support the idea that gut microbiota influence our cravings and mood. Our food cravings may actually be significantly shaped by the bacteria that we have inside our guts. Many gut bacteria can manufacture appetite-regulating peptide hormones and neuropeptides that regulate hunger. Some bacteria may even control our cravings through the production of the neurotransmitter dopamine. It doesn't take long for us to connect something sweet to our happiness, and a new craving has been established.

When it comes to mood, it appears that our microbes communicate with our brains through their production of short-chain fatty acids (SCFAs). When we eat fiber, some of our friendly *Bifido* bacteria consume the fiber and produce butyric acid as a by-product. Butyric acid is a short-chain fatty acid that repairs our gut lining but also reduces depression and sadness by encouraging the production of feel-good neurotransmitters.

If you have been struggling with chronic disease for a long time, supplements *might* help, but they are not required. And in many cases, I caution people to avoid the temptation to supplement their way to better health. With food, flavor compounds come from the nutritional context—minerals, vitamins, and antioxidants. When we artificially meet our nutritional needs by supplementing with pills and powders, we interfere with the natural flavor-nutrient feedback loop and deprive our bodies and our microbes of the complexity and innate intelligence that come from eating real food.

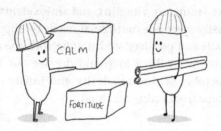

EXERCISE SETS THE MOOD

While exercise affects many aspects of health—both metabolic and mental—its least appreciated contribution may be to the plasticity of our gut microbes. The diverse and varied microbial community in the gut remains somewhat malleable throughout adult life—it can be influenced by lifestyle and environmental factors such as exercise, diet, and sleep.

When you are feeling healthy, relaxed, and safe, your gut flora generally work together harmoniously in a predictable, symbiotic manner. Oregon State University researchers found that when someone is under stress, his or her gut microbial communities become discombobulated and behave erratically, in ways that are unpredictable and vary from person to person.

Findings on how stress uniquely impacts your microbiome dovetail with many of the other findings cited in recent microbiome-gut-brain axis research. For example, researchers at Harvard Medical School reported that elite-level athletes who stayed calm, cool, and collected during stressful sports competitions shared common gut microbiome traits. The researchers believe there might be a correlation between mental toughness and the gut microbiome.

Finding ways to optimize well-being from the "bottom up" through nutrition or lifestyle, combined with a "top-down" approach that focuses on conscious ways to stimulate parasympathetic vagus nerve responses to inhibit "fight, flight, or freeze"—that is, to condition yourself to handle the stress response—may be a winning formula for maintaining microbiome symbiosis.

The sooner we get into the habit, the better, at least in terms of your microbes. Researchers out of the University of Colorado Boulder found that gut microorganisms are especially "plastic" at a young age. The animal study found that young rats who exercised voluntarily on a wheel every day developed robust and sophisticated microbial structures that included the expansion of probiotic bacterial species in their guts compared to both their sedentary counterparts and adult rats, even when the adult rats exercised as well.

We also know that there are many factors that reduce the variety of bacteria. These include antibiotics, artificial sweeteners, and even sugar! A decrease in diversity is associated with a variety of conditions, including diabetes, obesity, food and environmental allergies, and many inflammatory conditions. Research now points a positive light on movement by demonstrating a strong association between having a robust, healthy, and diverse set of gut bacteria and a person's level of cardiorespiratory fitness.

The lymphatic system moves lymph throughout the body, carrying both dead and alive bacteria that need to be removed along with it. Unlike the circulatory system, which has the heart to pump it, the lymphatic system is driven by motion, so it's essential for us to move our bodies to shuttle out bacteria that don't belong. Exercise may well be the best way to achieve that goal.

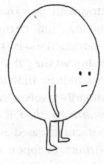
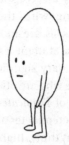

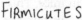
FIRMICUTES   BACTEROIDETES

A GOOD
NIGHT'S SLEEP

Our circadian rhythm is our 24-hour biological cycle, which governs our sleep-wake cycle. This rhythm of our sleep-wake pattern leads to fluctuations in the composition and function of our gut microbiota. In fact, all living organisms, including bacteria, have their own circadian rhythms that govern their biological function. Given that these cycles regulate and balance metabolic function in bacteria, chronically disrupted circadian rhythms caused by insufficient sleep can lead to metabolic dysfunction and gut dysbiosis in us. In other words, bacteria need rest, too. If our microbes don't sleep, we suffer the consequences.

The microbiome is not a stagnant entity; thousands of species are constantly competing with one another, negotiating with their host, evolving, and changing. Some species are more prevalent during the day, while others rise at night. Early evidence showed the gut microbiome to vary significantly between healthy individuals and those who are obese, which primarily involves higher numbers of *Firmicutes* over *Bacteroidetes*, or *the F/B ratio*. While Bacteroidetes also appear to fluctuate based on circadian rhythms, higher levels of Firmicutes appear to be more common in obese people and in mice. This ratio is not consistently connected to obesity in humans across all studies, but we can still fatten germ-free mice by loading them with microbes from an obese mouse or obese person. *Something* about these microbial communities affects body weight.

Scientists investigating the relationship between sleep and the microbiome have noted its effect on hormones that regulate sleep and wakefulness. Cortisol is critical to the sleep-wake cycle. This hormone plays a central role in our body's stress and inflammatory response cycle. When levels of cortisol rise in the morning, we feel energized and focused. Ideally, cortisol should drop in the evening in preparation for our sleep. Many types of gut microbes oscillate in activity and abundance throughout the day and night. For example, the gut microbe *Enterobacter aerogenes* is sensitive to melatonin, the sleep-signaling hormone. This bacteria is generally found in the gut and plays a role in fermenting sugars and producing gas but it can also cause opportunistic infections when spread to other tissues or when it overgrows due to antibiotic treatment. Melatonin is actually produced in the gut as well as the brain, and evidence suggests intestinal melatonin may operate on a different cyclical rhythm than the pineal melatonin generated in the brain.

Research suggests that following a consistent sleeping and eating rhythm can help restore healthy rhythms of gut microbial diversity. These microbial activity rhythms in turn help reset and maintain the circadian clock of cells in the intestinal wall and the liver. Just as the body's sleep patterns are regulated by different environmental cues—like light and darkness—our internal circadian clock also regulates other physiological functions, like digestion.

Toll-like receptors in the small intestine also follow a diurnal cycle, and they use our microbes to communicate with the intestinal wall and maintain consistent patterns of gastrointestinal functions. Animal studies conclude that as little as three months of disturbed circadian rhythms promotes increased intestinal permeability, also known as leaky gut. This can open the door, literally, to food allergies, inflammation, and other chronic symptoms.

Put very simply: our gut affects the quality of our sleep, and sleep affects the health and diversity of our microbiome. There is a strong connection between imbalance of gut microbes and stress, anxiety, depression, obesity and many inflammatory conditions, which in turn can trigger or exacerbate sleep disruptions.

Sweet dreams!

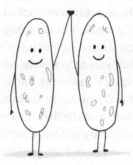

IT'S ABOUT RELATIONSHIPS

All relationships require time—lots of it. You and your microbiome are in it for the long haul. That means, when it comes to bringing your microbiome back to life after years of neglect and damage from antibiotics, over-the-counter medications, processed foods, stress, or even neglect, it's important not to approach it with a heavy hammer. Nor should you expect things to turn around for the better overnight.

Our ecosystem responds best to gentle and consistent nudges rather than drastic changes that occur all at once or randomly. It's not single actions, like taking a big dose of probiotics, or countless gut-healing protocols you might be advised to follow that make the most significant difference but the bacteria's *relationship* to you that ultimately shifts your inner terrain.

While our microbial communities ebb and flow, the activity of the strains and species present often remains the same. If they do change, we see focus shift to function. For example, a dominant lactic acid–producing strain of *Lactobacillus* in the vagina might suddenly disappear, but another lactic acid producer, perhaps a friendly strain of *Streptococcus*, might replace it. So although the species have changed, the same job still gets done. Different species can act in the same capacity. Whether it's a particular body part that houses the microbes or the type of species that is typically found in any one location of the body, it's more about how they act on our behalf than what labels we tend to assign to them. Like all things in nature, it's about working together and getting the job done.

Lactobacillus rhamnosus (*L. rhamnosus*) is a species of bacteria that has been shown to be useful for treating diarrhea, dermatitis, obesity, and food allergies, including allergies to peanuts and cow's milk. It's commonly found in familiar foods like yogurt, Parmigiano-Reggiano cheese, kefir, sausage, natto, as well as in certain probiotic supplements. In animal studies it was shown to reduce both anxiety and depression by increasing the levels of the neurotransmitter GABA. These benefits depend on the bacteria's ability to travel up and down the superhighway known as our vagus nerve, which runs from the gut to the brain. If the vagus nerve is severed, the effects disappear demonstrating an important partnership the bacteria have with the host.

L. rhamnosus can also alleviate obsessive-compulsive disorder (OCD) in mice. It appears to lower the levels of corticosteroids, which reduces levels of stress. It also produces a short-chain fatty acid called butyrate that heals the gut and penetrates the blood-brain barrier to act as an antidepressant. Another *Lactobacillus* species, *Lactobacillus plantarum* (*L. Plantarum*) is found in many fermented foods, including pickles, kimchi, sauerkraut, and brined olives. It has been shown in humans to mitigate soy allergies, enhance memory, and reduce inflammation. *L. plantarum* strains compete with other potentially pathogenic species like *Clostridium* and *Enterococcus* species, making it a good gut citizen to have on board.

People who struggle with chronic fatigue syndrome show less anxiety and improved gut health after consuming *Lactobacillus casei* (L. casei), which also enjoys the company of *Lactobacillus acidophilus*, both of which can be found in yogurt. Interestingly, *L. casei* causes the numbers of *Bifido* species to increase, which likely contributes to the positive effect—another example of how the bacteria are working synergistically in relationships on our behalf.

Our role is to respect and honor our relationship with our microbes and the shifts in our ecosystem, which will differ in response to our actions, environment, and lifestyle choices. To move things in our favor, we must be both patient and diligent as our bodies adjust. In fact, what you eat, but also *when* you eat, can drastically impact your health by changing the microbial communities in the gut. Fasting has a way of remodeling the gut microbiome toward a healthier community profile.

In Part II, I talked about "pressing pause," or fasting, to give the digestive system a rest. I like to think of fasting as the "no-till" approach used in farming. No-till farming, a type of soil conservation farming, prepares the land for farming without mechanically disturbing the soil. Because the soil is not being frequently agitated, no-till farming promotes biodiversity in and around the soil. Organisms like mycorrhizal fungi, which make beneficial associations with crop roots and earthworms, increase the water retention of the soil and are allowed to flourish through the no-till approach. When we allow our microbial community to "rest," we too create an opportunity for the good microbes to work together and flourish. We know many species of "bad" bacteria have a relatively short doubling time compared to our commensal good bacteria, so if we fast, they will tend to starve more quickly than the healthy bacteria in the gut.

Historically, our bacteria had to survive in conditions with far less food, which means that when we give them too much too often, they likely overdo it. Surprisingly, periods of intermittent fasting seem to flip the "growth switch" for the good guys. When we fast, we increase two of our most important keystone "protective" strains of bacteria, *Akkermansia muciniphila* and *Faecalibacterium prausnitzii*, both of which have been associated with reducing inflammation. These keystone bacteria are considered important for human health and may be key factors in combating chronic disease because antibiotics, stress, poor diet, glyphosate exposure, and other environmental toxins seem to easily diminish their populations in our guts.

It's clear that we benefit from our microbes. Assuming we treat them right, our microbes can live in symbiosis with us and benefit as well.

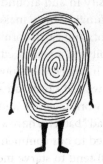

You are unique

CONNECTING THE DOTS

Today, over half of the world's population is afflicted with some form of chronic disease. People who die from chronic disease lose, on average, one-third of their living years. Think about that—losing one-third of your life to a *completely preventable* disease.

As I have said many times throughout this book, chronic disease is preventable, and if you have it, it's reversible. We have become so complacent to the early warning signs and patterns of chronic disease that we are forced to react to it only once the disease has declared its presence. Oftentimes it can be easy to look at cases where other people have experienced a life-changing event, sometimes tragic, that forced them to reconstruct their lives and simply admire them for getting it all figured out. But I'm asking you to recognize your capacity to heal. We all hold the same power to change. Healing is not for the select few.

Many, if not all, of today's illnesses and chronic diseases involve the microbiome. This isn't a new discovery, but it's underappreciated and most certainly an underutilized approach in optimizing health. We can no longer assume that pills will solve our health problems, and we know for sure they do not cure chronic disease.

No two microbiomes are the same—we are all unique. We all tend to share a lot of the same types of microbes, but it appears that we, the hosts, personalize how the bacteria behave. Even in sets of twins, microbes seem to diverge over time. The uniqueness of you makes it critical to have your own affirming beliefs and consistent healthy behaviors to shift your inner ecosystem toward optimizing health. When it comes to your health, there is *no one-size-fits-all approach*. You are your own healer, and your microbes are your allies in regenerating health.

You must take the responsibility for your health by making the lifestyle changes that I have outlined here in this book: honoring your values, tapping into the nutritional intelligence of your food, reclaiming the power of sleep, cooking more, mastering your attention, reconnecting with nature, and partnering with your microbial allies. On every level, when you move forward in a positive direction with simple, consistent changes, you are regenerating health and moving away from disease.

When I set out to write this book, initially titled *Resilience*, I was determined to answer the question: *What truly conditions the body to overcome chronic illness?* What I discovered is that chronic disease is complex. How you got here is unique to you. How you unravel your illness is also unique to you. There are so many layers of illness today, making it more and more difficult for anyone to figure out what's wrong. And most important, it's not your fault. It does, however, require you to ask yourself big questions before you make small changes. I can't do that for you, but my hope is that this book opens that door in your mind and your heart so that you can start having those conversations with yourself, at your table, and in your life with others.

I have always felt that the topics of growth mind-set, lifestyle habits, and even microbes circled around improving human health and that there was a relevant link to planetary health. I've researched these topics and read countless books that tackle these important subjects in depth. *End Chronic Disease* does not aim to unpack these subjects in depth but rather aims to invite you to consider them in your own life and their connection to your health. Inspired by the simplicity and practical advice of Michael Pollan's *Food Rules: An Eater's Manual*, I wanted to link them together with our capacity to end chronic disease and adapt to change.

Changing your lifestyle is going to require you do things that feel like hard work, but all of them are simple. Caring for yourself is part of caring for the environment. We are all part of a larger whole—a complex, living ecosystem. It just takes practice to create a new way of thinking and doing things. Once you connect the dots to the healing power of your beliefs, behaviors, and bacteria and their interconnectedness to the health of the planet, together, we can *End Chronic Disease*!

AFTERWORD

You may still be thinking, but how? What does healing from chronic disease actually look like in everyday life, exactly? Tell me what to eat. Tell me what to do. Tell me what to avoid. I want to know specifically what you did. Trust me, I understand the desire to want everything mapped out. We all want the solutions to be clear and straightforward. My resistance to addressing these points with a specific set of instructions is because for so long I followed the *rules* laid out by others and it never translated to long-term health. Instead the rules became a burden.

"Dis-*ease*" happens when the body is pushed out of balance and there is rarely, if ever, a single cause for this imbalance. The complexity of how each of us arrives at the place of chronic disease is why there is *no one size fits all approach* to healing. That said, there are multiple ways to heal and it looks different for everyone. There are countless resources on how to eat clean, let go of anger, move more, and nourish our microbiome. I've written articles and lectured on these topics, and I teach courses that outline the functional approach to regenerating health. Of course, many people need the support of others and I'm not suggesting anyone go it alone. The expertise of others, including the use of supplements, medications, therapies or other treatments can be life-changing at various stages on your healing journey. However, I strongly believe that focusing on the intelligence of the whole is far more empowering than being categorized into certain diseases only to be managed with a certain dietary approach or treatment.

Perhaps, you are willing to accept that masking symptoms or a dependency on pharmaceutical drugs is not true healing. But, we must be careful not to let the pendulum swing too far in any direction. Obsessing over health-promoting practices or nutraceuticals in response to the fear of disease, bacteria, or toxins is also unhealthy.

Ultimately, regenerating health is about creating a new pattern, a rhythm for your life. It's not a rigorous list of things you need to do every day. I want to emphasize that when you take ownership of your beliefs, behaviors, and bacteria, you are flipping the model of care to one in which you hold the power to heal.

After all, do we want to pass down supplemental protocols and restrictive diets to our children? I know I don't. The legacy I want to leave my children and the next generation is not going to be how to "cleanse heavy metals" or "rebalance bacterial dysbiosis." I want them to know nature through the act of cooking and caring for themselves—that spices can be strongly antimicrobial without being anti-life and that without sufficient physical activity, they will find it difficult to make progress in health, regardless of how good their food may be. They will know through their senses that there is no food quite as comforting and emblematic of home as soup. Much like we model kindness to our children, health is something that we tend to gently in our daily lives without rigidity. Health is woven into our daily life seamlessly.

As you are moving away from disease and toward health you want to learn *how to think* versus *what to think*. This allows you to replicate different methods as needed for yourself and others. But more importantly, it also allows you to modify factors for different situations, which provides you the flexibility to care for and teach others. This is individualized, personalized care.

You deserve to be the master of your own health with the capacity to pass down nutritional wisdom and lifestyle behaviors that are grounded in optimizing health versus the fear of disease.

My mission is to change the way we "treat" chronic disease by first modeling a different way of resolving it and then educating you how to do the same. This is my greatest desire—to help you reignite the innate intelligence you were born with. In fact, much like nature, the body prefers inner intelligence over outside influences. Let's go inside ourselves, together.

SELECTED BIBLIOGRAPHY

Introduction

Bland, Jeffrey. *The Disease Delusion: Conquering the Causes of Chronic Illness for a Healthier, Longer, and Happier Life.* New York: Harper Wave, 2015.

Collen, Alanna. *10% Human: How Your Body's Microbes Hold the Key to Health and Happiness.* New York: HarperCollins, 2016.

Marano, Hara Estroff. "The Art of Resilience." *Psychology Today*, May 1, 2003. http://www.psychologytoday.com/us/articles/200305/the-art-resilience.

PART I: BELIEFS

Cook, Gareth. "The Science of Healing Thoughts." *Scientific American*, January 19, 2016. http://www.scientificamerican.com/article/the-science-of-healing-thoughts/.

Values

Rubin, Beverly S. "Bisphenol A: An Endocrine Disruptor with Widespread Exposure and Multiple Effects." *The Journal of Steroid Biochemistry and Molecular Biology* 127, nos. 1–2 (October 2011): 27–34. https://doi.org/10.1016/j.jsbmb.2011.05.002.

Wisdom

Douillard, John. *Eat Wheat: A Scientific and Clinically-Proven Approach to Safely Bringing Wheat and Dairy Back into Your Diet.* New York: Morgan James, 2017.

Thom, Dickson. *Bioregulatory Medicine: An Innovative Holistic Approach to Self-Healing*. White River Junction, VT: Chelsea Green, 2018.

Nourishment

Bureau, Janice L., and Rodney J. Bushway. "HPLC Determination of Carotenoids in Fruits and Vegetables in the United States." *Journal of Food Science* 51, no. 1 (January 1986): 128–30. https://doi.org/10.1111/j.1365-2621.1986.tb10851.x.

Graham, Robin D., Ross M. Welch, and Howarth E. Bouis. "Addressing Micronutrient Malnutrition through Enhancing the Nutritional Quality of Staple Foods: Principles, Perspectives and Knowledge Gaps." *Advances in Agronomy* 70 (2001): 77–142. https://doi.org/10.1016/s0065-2113(01)70004-1.

Hanson, Peter M., Ray-yu Yang, Jane Wu, Jen-tzu Chen, Dolores Ledesma, and Samson C. S. Tsou. "Variation for Antioxidant Activity and Antioxidants in Tomato." *Journal of the American Society for Horticultural Science* 129, no. 5 (2004): 704–11. https://doi.org/10.21273/jashs.129.5.0704.

Herz, Rachel. *Why You Eat What You Eat: The Science behind Our Relationship with Food*. New York: W. W. Norton, 2018.

Ju, Songwen, Jingyao Mu, Terje Dokland, Xiaoying Zhuang, Qilong Wang, Hong Jiang, Xiaoyu Xiang, et al. "Grape Exosome-like Nanoparticles Induce Intestinal Stem Cells and Protect Mice From DSS-Induced Colitis." *Molecular Therapy* 21, no. 7 (July 2013): 1345–57. https://doi.org/10.1038/mt.2013.64.

Schatzker, Mark. *The Dorito Effect: The Surprising New Truth about Food and Flavor*. New York: Simon & Schuster, 2015.

Semba, Richard D. "Nutrition and Development: A Historical Perspective." In *Nutrition and Health in a Developing World*, 3rd ed., edited by Saskia de Pee, Douglas Taren, and Martin W. Bloem, 3–29. New York: Humana, 2017. https://doi.org/10.1007/978-3-319-43739-2_1.

Sherman, Paul W., and Jennifer Billing. "Darwinian Gastronomy: Why We Use Spices; Spices Taste Good Because They Are Good for Us." *BioScience* 49, no. 6 (June 1999): 453–63. https://doi.org/10.2307/1313553.

"Syrup Science." The website for the University of Rhode Island. Accessed August 28, 2019. http://www.uri.edu/features/syrup-science/.

Teng, Yun, et al. "Plant-Derived Exosomal MicroRNAs Shape Gut Microbiota." Cell Host & Microbe, vol 24., no. 5, 2018, doi:10.1016/j.chom.

Ventura, Alison K., and Julie A. Mennella. "Innate and Learned Preferences for Sweet Taste during Childhood." *Current Opinion in Clinical Nutrition and Metabolic Care* 14, no. 4 (July 2011): 379–84. https://doi.org/10.1097/mco.0b013e328346df65.

Intuition

Day, Laura. *Practical Intuition: How to Harness the Power of Your Instinct and Make It Work for You.* New York: Broadway Books, 1997.

Lufityanto, Galang, Chris Donkin, and Joel Pearson. "Measuring Intuition: Nonconscious Emotional Information Boosts Decision Accuracy and Confidence." *Psychological Science* 27, no. 5 (May 2016): 622–34. https://doi.org/10.1177/0956797616629403.

Zukav, Gary. *The Seat of the Soul.* New York: Simon & Schuster, 1989.

Emotions

Dekker, Jacqueline M., Evert G. Schouten, Peter Klootwijk, Jan Pool, Cees A. Swenne, and Daan Kromhout. "Heart Rate Variability from Short Electrocardiographic Recordings Predicts Mortality from All Causes in Middle-Aged and Elderly Men: The Zutphen Study." *American Journal of Epidemiology* 145, no. 10 (May 15, 1997): 899–908. https://doi.org/10.1093/oxfordjournals.aje.a009049.

Dispenza, Joe. *Becoming Supernatural: How Common People Are Doing the Uncommon.* Carlsbad, CA: Hay House, 2017.

Friedman, Howard S., and Stephanie Booth-Kewley. "The 'Disease-Prone Personality': A Meta-Analytic View of the Construct," *American Psychologist* 42, no. 6 (June 1987): 539–55.

Goleman, Daniel. *Emotional Intelligence*. New York: Random House, 2005.

Nelson, Bradley. *The Emotion Code: How to Release Your Trapped Emotions for Abundant Health, Love, and Happiness*. Mesquite, NV: Wellness Unmasked Publishing, 2007.

Tozzi, Paolo. "Does Fascia Hold Memories?" *Journal of Bodywork and Movement Therapies* 18, no. 2 (2014): 259–65. https://doi.org/10.1016/j.jbmt.2013.11.010.

Connection

Agrawal, Radha. *Belong: Find Your People, Create Community, and Live a More Connected Life*. New York: Workman, 2018.

Provenza, Frederick D. *Nourishment: What Animals Can Teach Us about Rediscovering Our Nutritional Wisdom*. White River Junction, VT: Chelsea Green, 2018.

Provenza, Frederick D., Scott L. Kronberg, and Pablo Gregorini. "Is Grassfed Meat and Dairy Better for Human and Environmental Health?" *Frontiers in Nutrition* 6 (March 2019). https://doi.org/10.3389/fnut.2019.00026.

"The Global Risks Report 2018." World Economic Forum. January 17, 2018. http://www.weforum.org/reports/the-global-risks-report-2018.

Tickell, Josh. *Kiss the Ground: How the Food You Eat Can Reverse Climate Change, Heal Your Body, and Ultimately Save Our World*. New York: Enliven, 2018.

"Toxic Secret: Pesticides Uncovered in Store Brand Cereal, Beans, Produce." Friends of the Earth. Accessed July 21, 2019. foe.org/food-testing-results/.

PART II: BEHAVIORS

Eat on the Wild Side

Blair, Katrina. *The Wild Wisdom of Weeds: 13 Essential Plants for Human Survival*. White River Junction, VT: Chelsea Green, 2014.

Hites, Ronald A., Jeffery A. Foran, David O. Carpenter, M. Coreen Hamilton, Barbara A. Knuth, and Steven J. Schwager. "Global Assessment of Organic Contaminants in Farmed Salmon." *Science* 303, no. 5655 (January 2004): 226–29. https://doi.org/10.1126/science.1091447.

Isokauppila, Tero. *Healing Mushrooms: A Practical and Culinary Guide to Using Mushrooms for Whole Body Health*. New York: Penguin, 2017.

Smits, Samuel A., Jeff Leach, Erica D. Sonnenburg, Carlos G. Gonzalez, Joshua S. Lichtman, Gregor Reid, Rob Knight, et al. "Seasonal Cycling in the Gut Microbiome of the Hadza Hunter-Gatherers of Tanzania." *Science* 357, no. 6353 (August 2017): 802–6. https://doi.org/10.1126/science.aan4834.

Master Your Attention

Alter, Adam. *Irresistible: The Rise of Addictive Technology and the Business of Keeping Us Hooked*. New York: Penguin, 2018.

Turkle, Sherry. *Reclaiming Conversation: The Power of Talk in a Digital Age*. New York: Penguin, 2016.

Learn to Breathe

Barelli, Pat A. "Nasopulmonary Physiology." In *Behavioral and Psychological Approaches to Breathing Disorders*, edited by Beverly H. Timmons and Ronald Ley, 47–57. New York: Springer, 1994. https://doi.org/10.1007/978-1-4757-9383-3_3.

Bhasin, Manoj K., Jeffery A. Dusek, Bei-Hung Chang, Marie G. Joseph, John W. Denninger, Gregory L. Fricchione, Herbert Benson, and Towia A. Libermann. "Relaxation

Response Induces Temporal Transcriptome Changes in Energy Metabolism, Insulin Secretion and Inflammatory Pathways." *PLOS ONE* 8, no. 5 (May 2013). https://doi.org/10.1371/journal.pone.0062817.

Shannahoff-Khalsa, David. "The Ultradian Rhythm of Alternating Cerebral Hemispheric Activity." *International Journal of Neuroscience* 70, no. 3–4 (1993): 285–98. https://doi.org/10.3109/00207459309000583.

Reclaim the Power of Sleep

Broussard, Josiane L., and Eve Van Cauter. "Disturbances of Sleep and Circadian Rhythms: Novel Risk Factors for Obesity." *Current Opinion in Endocrinology & Diabetes and Obesity* 23, no. 5 (October 2016): 353–59. https://doi.org/10.1097/med.0000000000000276.

Eimer, William A., Deepak Kumar Vijaya Kumar, Nanda Kumar N. Shanmugam, Kevin J. Washicosky, Alex S. Rodriguez, Bence György, Xandra O. Breakefield, Rudolph E. Tanzi, and Robert D. Moir. "Alzheimer's Disease-Associated -amyloid Is Rapidly Seeded by *herpesviridae* to Protect Against Brain Infection." *SSRN Electronic Journal* (2018). https://doi.org/10.2139/ssrn.3155923.

Irwin, M., J. McClintick, C. Costlow, M. Fortner, J. White, and J. C. Gillin. "Partial Night Sleep Deprivation Reduces Natural Killer and Cellular Immune Responses in Humans." *The FASEB Journal* 10, no. 5 (April 1996): 643–53. https://doi.org/10.1096/fasebj.10.5.8621064.

Louveau, Antoine, Benjamin A. Plog, Salli Antila, Kari Alitalo, Maiken Nedergaard, and Jonathan Kipnis. "Understanding the Functions and Relationships of the Glymphatic System and Meningeal Lymphatics." *The Journal of Clinical Investigation* 127, no. 9 (September 2017): 3210–19. https://doi.org/10.1172/jci90603.

Paulose, Jiffin K., John M. Wright, Akruti G. Patel, Vincent M. Cassone. "Human Gut Bacteria Are Sensitive to Melatonin and Express Endogenous Circadian Rhythmicity." *PLOS ONE* 11, no. 1 (January 2016): e0146643. https://doi.org/10.1371/journal.pone.0146643.

Soscia, Stephanie J., James E. Kirby, Kevin J. Washicosky, Stephanie M. Tucker, Martin Ingelsson, Bradley Hyman, Mark A. Burton, et al. "The Alzheimer's Disease-Associated Amyloid -Protein Is an Antimicrobial Peptide." *PLOS ONE* 5, no. 3 (March 2010): e9505 https://doi.org/10.1371/journal.pone.0009505.

Walker, Matthew P. *Why We Sleep: The New Science of Sleep and Dreams*. New York: Penguin, 2018.

Protect Your Microbial Allies

Becattini, Simone, Ying Taur, and Eric G. Palmer. "Antibiotic-Induced Changes in the Intestinal Microbiota and Disease." *Trends in Molecular Medicine* 22, no. 6 (June 2016): 458–78.

Bordenstein, Seth R., and Kevin R. Theis. "Host Biology in Light of the Microbiome: Ten Principles of Holobionts and Hologenomes." *PLOS Biology* 13, no. 8 (August 2015): e1002226. https://doi.org/10.1371/journal.pbio.1002226.

Francino, M. P., and A. Moya. "Effects of Antibiotic Use on the Microbiota of the Gut and Associated Alterations of Immunity and Metabolism." *EMJ Gastroenterology* 1 (2013): 74–80.

Hegarty, James W., Caitriona M. Guinane, R. Paul Ross, Colin Hill, and Paul D. Cotter. "Bacteriocin Production: A Relatively Unharnessed Probiotic Trait?" *F1000Research* 5, no. 2587 (October 2016). https://doi.org/10.12688/f1000research.9615.1.

Simplify

Becker, Joshua. *The More of Less: Finding the Life You Want under Everything You Own*. Colorado Springs: WaterBrook, 2016

Kondo, Marie. *The Life-Changing Magic of Tidying Up: The Japanese Art of Decluttering and Organizing*. Berkeley: Ten Speed, 2016..

Pelley, Janet. "Dust, Unsettled." *ACS Central Science* 3, no. 1 (2017): 5–9. https://doi.org/10.1021/acscentsci.7b00006.

Redefine Stress

Foster, Jane A., Linda Rinaman, and John F. Cryan. "Stress and the Gut-Brain Axis: Regulation by the Microbiome." *Neurobiology of Stress* 7 (December 2017): 124–36. https://doi.org/10.1016/j.ynstr.2017.03.001.

Lima-Ojeda, Juan M., Rainer Rupprecht, and Thomas C. Baghai. "'I Am I and My Bacterial Circumstances': Linking Gut Microbiome, Neurodevelopment, and Depression." *Frontiers in Psychiatry* 8 (August 2017): 153. https://doi.org/10.3389/fpsyt.2017.00153.

Marini, Ann, Margherita Popolo, Hongna Pan, Nicolas Blondeau, and Robert H. Lipsky. "Brain Adaptation to Stressful Stimuli: A New Perspective on Potential Therapeutic Approaches Based on BDNF and NMDA Receptors." *CNS & Neurological Disorders: Drug Targets* 7, no. 4 (2008): 382–90. https://doi.org/10.2174/187152708786441849.

Weaver, Ian, C. G., et al. "Epigenetic Programming by Maternal Behavior." *Nature Neuroscience* 7, no. 8 (2004): 847–54. doi:10.1038/nn1276.

Zaneveld, Jesse R., Ryan McMinds, and Rebecca Vega Thurber. "Stress and Stability: Applying the Anna Karenina Principle to Animal Microbiomes." *Nature Microbiology* 2, no. 9 (2017): 17121. https://doi.org/10.1038/nmicrobiol.2017.121.

Move Your Body Often

Bowman, Katy. *Movement Matters*. Sequim, WA: Propriometrics, 2016

Estaki, Mehrbod, Jason Pither, Peter Baumeister, Jonathan P. Little, Sandeep K. Gil, Sanjoy Ghosh, Zahra Ahmadi-Vand, Katelyn R. Marsden, and Deanna L. Gibson. "Cardiorespiratory Fitness as a Predictor of Intestinal Microbial Diversity and Distinct Metagenomic Functions." *Microbiome* 4 (2016): 42. https://doi.org/10.1186/s40168-016-0189-7.

Sleiman, Sama F., Jeffrey Henry, Rami Al-Haddad, Lauretta El Hayek, Edwina Abou Haidar, Thomas Stringer, Devyani

Ulja, et al. "Exercise Promotes the Expression of Brain Derived Neurotrophic Factor (BDNF) through the Action of the Ketone Body -Hydroxybutyrate." *ELife* 5 (2016): e15092. https://doi.org/10.7554/elife.15092.

Pick Three

García, Héctor, and Francesc Miralles. *Ikigai: The Japanese Secret to a Long and Happy Life*. Waterville: Thorndike, 2018.

Cook Your Own Food

Gibbs, Nancy. "The Magic of the Family Meal." *TIME*, June 4, 2006. http://content.time.com/time/magazine/article/0,9171,1200760,00.html.

Have Faith

Bullard, Gabe. "The World's Newest Major Religion: No Religion." *National Geographic*, April 22, 2016. http://news.nationalgeographic.com/2016/04/160422-atheism-agnostic-secular-nones-rising-religion/.

Chittister, Joan. *The Time Is Now: A Call to Uncommon Courage*. New York: Convergent, 2019.

Lucchetti, Giancarlo, Alessandra L. G. Lucchetti, and Harold G. Koenig. "Impact of Spirituality/Religiosity on Mortality: Comparison with Other Health Interventions." *Explore* 7, no. 4 (July–August 2011): 234–38. https://doi.org/10.1016/j.explore.2011.04.005.

Newberg, Andrew B. "The Neuroscientific Study of Spiritual Practices." *Frontiers in Psychology* 5 (March 2014): 215. https://doi.org/10.3389/fpsyg.2014.00215.

Parnia, Sam, and Peter Fenwick. "Near Death Experiences in Cardiac Arrest: Visions of a Dying Brain or Visions of a New Science of Consciousness." *Resuscitation* 52, no. 1 (January 2002): 5–11. https://doi.org/10.1016/s0300-9572(01)00469-5.

Tiffany, Demke. Review of *Principles of Neurotheology*, by Andrew B. Newberg. *Zygon* 46, no. 3 (September 2011): 763–64. https://doi.org/10.1111/j.1467-9744.2011.01211.x.

Connect with Nature

Arvay, Clemens G. *The Biophilia Effect: A Scientific and Spiritual Exploration of the Healing Bond between Humans and Nature*. Louisville: Sounds True, 2018.

Cho, Kyoung Sang, Young-ran Lim, Kyungho Lee, Jaeseok Lee, Jang Ho Lee, and Im-Soon Lee. "Terpenes from Forests and Human Health." *Toxicological Research* 33, no. 2 (April 2017): 97–106.

Gershenzon, Jonathan, and Natalia Dudareva. "The Function of Terpene Natural Products in the Natural World." *Nature Chemical Biology* 3 (2007): 408–14. https://doi.org/10.1038/nchembio.2007.5.

Kim, In-Hee, Chan Kim, Kayeon Seong, Myung-Haeng Hur, Heon Man Lim, and Myeong Soo Lee. "Essential Oil Inhalation on Blood Pressure and Salivary Cortisol Levels in Prehypertensive and Hypertensive Subjects." *Evidence-Based Complementary and Alternative Medicine* 2012 (2012): 984203.

Li, Q., K. Morimoto, A. Nakadai, H. Inagaki, M. Katsumata, T. Shimizu, Y. Hirata, et al. "Forest Bathing Enhances Human Natural Killer Activity and Expression of Anti-Cancer Proteins." *International Journal of Immunopathology and Pharmacology* 20, no. 2 (April 2007): 3–8. https://doi.org/10.1177/03946320070200s202.

Lohr, Virginia I. "Benefits of Nature: What We Are Learning about Why People Respond to Nature." *Journal of Physiological Anthropology* 26, no. 2 (April 2007): 83–85.

Matthews, D. M., and Jenks, S. M. "Ingestion of Mycobacterium vaccae Decreases Anxiety-related Behavior and Improves Learning in Mice." *Behavioural Processes* 96 (2013): 27–35.

Selhub, Eva M., and Alan C. Logan. *Your Brain on Nature: The Science of Nature's Influence on Your Health, Happiness, and Vitality*. New York: HarperCollins, 2014.

Wilson, E. O. "Biophilia and the Conservation Ethic," in *The Biophilia Hypothesis*, edited by S. R. Kellert and E. O. Wilson, 31–41. Washington, DC: Island, 1993.

Press Pause

Longo, Valter D. "Fasting, Circadian Rhythms, and Time-Restricted Feeding in Healthy Lifespan." *Cell Metabolism* 23, no. 6 (June 14, 2016): 1048–59. http://dx.doi.org/10.1016/j.cmet.2016.06.00.

———. *The Longevity Diet: Discover the New Science behind Stem Cell Activation and Regeneration to Slow Aging, Fight Disease, and Optimize Weight.* New York: Avery, 2018.

Luders, Eileen, Florian Kurth, Emeran A. Mayer, Arthur W. Toga, Katherine L. Narr, and Christian Gaser. "The Unique Brain Anatomy of Meditation Practitioners: Alterations in Cortical Gyrification." *Frontiers in Human Neuroscience* 6 (February 2012): 34. https://doi.org/10.3389/fnhum.2012.00034.

Honor Your Transitions

Beck, Renee, and Sydney Barbara Metrick. *The Art of Ritual.* Berkeley: Apocryphile, 2009.

Broadbent, Elizabeth, Jan W. Schoones, Jitske Tiemensma, and Ad A. Kapstein. "A Systematic Review of Patients' Drawing of Illness: Implications for Research Using the Common Sense Model." *Health Psychology Review* (December 2018). https://doi.org/10.1080/17437199.2018.1558088.

Take Action

Lelic, Dina, Imran Khan Niazi, Kelly Holt, Mads Jochumsen, Kim Dremstrup, Paul Yielder, Bernadette Murphy, Asbjørn Mohr Drewes, and Heidi Haavik. "Manipulation of Dysfunctional Spinal Joints Affects Sensorimotor Integration in the Prefrontal Cortex: A Brain Source Localization Study." *Neural Plasticity* 2016 (2016): 3704964. https://doi.org/10.1155/2016/3704964.

Part III: Bacteria

David, Lawrence A., Corinne F. Maurice, Rachel N. Carmo-
dy, David B. Gootenberg, Julie E. Button, Benjamin E.
Wolfe, Alisha V. Ling, et al. "Diet Rapidly and Repro-
ducibly Alters the Human Gut Microbiome." *Nature*
505, no. 7484 (2013): 559–63. https://doi.org/10.1038/
nature12820.

Dietert, Rodney. *The Human Superorganism: How the Microbiome Is Revolutionizing the Pursuit of a Healthy Life.* New
York: Dutton, 2016.

Moise, Ana Maria R. *The Gut Microbiome: Exploring the Connection between Microbes, Diet, and Health.* Santa Barbara:
Greenwood, 2017.

Setting the Stage: First 1,000 Days

Gensollen, Thomas, Shankar S. Iyer, Dennis L. Kasper, and
Richard S. Blumberg. "How Colonization by Microbiota in Early Life Shapes the Immune System." *Science*
352, no. 6285 (April 29, 2016): 539–44. https://doi.
org/10.1126/science.aad9378.

Harman, Toni, and Alex Wakeford. *Your Baby's Microbiome:
The Critical Role of Vaginal Birth and Breastfeeding for Life-
long Health.* White River Junction: Chelsea Green, 2017.

Horton, Daniel B., Frank I. Scott, Kevin Haynes, Mary E.
Putt, Carlos D. Rose, James D. Lewis, and Brian L. Storm.
"Antibiotic Exposure and Juvenile Idiopathic Arthritis: A
Case-Control Study." *Pediatrics* 136, no. 2 (August 2015):
e333–43. https://doi.org/10.1542/peds.2015-0036d.

Perlmutter, David, and Kristin Loberg. *Brain Maker: The Power
of Gut Microbes to Heal and Protect Your Brain—for Life.*
New York: Little, Brown, 2015.

Wampach, Linda, Anna Heintz-Buschart, Joëlle V. Fritz, Javier
Ramiro-Garcia, Janine Habier, Malte Herold, Shaman
Narayanasamy, et al. "Birth Mode Is Associated with
Earliest Strain-Conferred Gut Microbiome Functions and
Immunostimulatory Potential." *Nature Communications*

9 (2018): 5019. https://doi.org/10.1038/s41467-018-07631-x.

Biodiversity Is Key

Eckburg, P. B., Elisabeth M. Bik, Charles N. Bernstein, Elizabeth Purdom, Les Dethlefsen, Michael Sargent, Steven R. Gill, Karen E. Nelson, and David A. Relman. "Diversity of the Human Intestinal Microbial Flora." *Science* 308, no. 5728 (June 10, 2005): 1635–38. https://doi.org/10.1126/science.1110591.

Prescott, Susan L., and Alan C. Logan. *The Secret Life of Your Microbiome: Why Nature and Biodiversity Are Essential to Health and Happiness*. Gabriola Island: New Society, 2017.

Valdes, Ana M., Jens Walter, Eran Segal, and Tim D. Spector. "Role of the Gut Microbiota in Nutrition and Health." *BMJ* 261, supp. 1 (2018): 36–44. https://doi.org/10.1136/bmj.k2179.

Yong, Ed. *I Contain Multitudes: The Microbes within Us and a Grander View of Life*. New York: Ecco, 2018.

Reconnect

Taheri, M., S. M. J. Mortazavi, M. Moradi, S. Mansouri, G. R. Hatam, and F. Nouri. "Evaluation of the Effect of Radiofrequency Radiation Emitted from Wi-Fi Router and Mobile Phone Simulator on the Antibacterial Susceptibility of Pathogenic Bacteria *Listeria monocytogenes* and *Escherichia coli*." *Dose-Response* 15, no. 1 (January–March 2017): 1–8. https://doi.org/10.1177/1559325816688527.

Vasistha, Sharsti, and Akshay Garg. "Effect of Electromagnetic Radiation on *Lactobacillus* Species." *Journal of Chemical and Pharmaceutical Research* 8, no. 7 (2016): 123–26.

Yalçınkaya, Burak, Aytül Sofu, Özlem Co kun, and Selçuk Çömlekçi. "Effect of 2.45 GHz Electromagnetic Radiation on Evolution of *Lactobacillus rhamnosus*." *2014 18th National Biomedical Engineering Meeting* (2014). https://doi.org/10.1109/biyomut.2014.7026380.

Everything Has a Purpose

Dan, Jennifer M., Colin Havenar-Daughton, Kayla Kendric, Rita Al-kolla, Kirti Kaushik, Sandy L. Rosales, Ericka L. Anderson, et al. "Recurrent Group A Streptococcus Tonsillitis Is an Immunosusceptibility Disease Involving Antibody Deficiency and Aberrant T_{FH} Cells." *Science Translational Medicine* 11, no. 478 (February 6, 2019): eaau3776. https://doi.org/10.1126/scitranslmed.aau3776.

Duke University Medical Center. "Evolution of the Human Appendix: A Biological 'Remnant' No More." *ScienceDaily*, August 21, 2009.

Immunity

Deshpande DA, Wang WCH, McIlmoyle EL, Robinett KS, Schillinger RM, An SS, Sham JSK, Liggett SB. "Bitter taste receptors on airway smooth muscle bronchodialate by localized calcium signaling and reverse obstruction." Natural Medicine. Published online October 24, 2010.

Freund, Jenna R., and Robert J. Lee. "Taste Receptors in the Upper Airway." *World Journal of Otorhinolaryngology—Head and Neck Surgery* 4, no. 1 (March 2018): 67–76. https://doi.org/10.1016/j.wjorl.2018.02.004.

Perelman School of Medicine at the University of Pennsylvania. "Bitter Taste Receptors Regulate Upper Respiratory Defense System." *ScienceDaily*, October 8, 2012.

Built-In Apothecary

Anderson, Scott C., John F. Cryan, and Ted Dinan. *The Psychobiotic Revolution: Mood, Food, and the New Science of the Gut-Brain Connection.* Washington, DC: National Geographic, 2017.

LeBlanc, Jean Guy, Christian Milani, Graciela Savoy de Giori, Fernando Sesma, Douwe van Sinderen, and Marco Ventura. "Bacteria as Vitamin Suppliers to Their Host: A Gut Microbiota Perspective." *Current Opinion in Biotechnology* 24, no. 2 (April 2013): 160–68. https://doi.org/10.1016/j.copbio.2012.08.005.

Exercise Sets the Mood

Mailing, Lucy J., Jacob Allen, Thomas Buford, Christopher Fields, and Jeffrey Woods. "Exercise and the Gut Microbiome: A Review of the Evidence, Potential Mechanisms, and Implications for Human Health." *Exercise and Sport Sciences Reviews* 47, no. 2 (April 2019): 75–85. https://doi.org/10.1249/jes.0000000000000183.

A Good Night's Sleep

Dijk, Derk-Jan. "Sleep, Rhythms and Metabolism: Too Many Links to Be Ignored." *Journal of Sleep Research* 25, no. 4 (2016): 379–80. https://doi.org/10.1111/jsr.12449.

Liang, Xue, and Garret A. FitzGerald. "Timing the Microbes: The Circadian Rhythm of the Gut Microbiome." *Journal of Biological Rhythms* 32, no. 6 (2017): 505–515. https://doi.org/10.1177/0748730417729066.

It's about Relationships

van Passel, Mark W. J., Ravi Kant, Erwin G. Zoetendal, Caroline M. Plugge, Muriel Derrien, Stephanie A. Malfatti, Patrick S. G. Chain, et al. "The Genome of *Akkermansia muciniphila*, a Dedicated Intestinal Mucin Degrader, and Its Use in Exploring Intestinal Metagenomes." *PLOS ONE* 6, no. 3 (March 2011): e16876. https://doi.org/10.1371/journal.pone.0016876.

ACKNOWLEDGMENTS

This book represents the efforts and influence of many. First and foremost, thank you to all of the people who have courageously changed their lives, reversed their chronic disease, and taught me the most about how people heal—proving that our choices matter. My family is among this brave group, and I am proud to say that we successfully reversed over 20 chronic diseases collectively in our family of five through the healing power of our beliefs, behaviors, and bacteria.

There are no words to adequately thank my husband, Stephen. I owe him a great deal of gratitude not only for serving as the co-pilot on our healing journey but for reading countless drafts of my manuscript and offering meaningful suggestions as well as taking on more of the picks-ups, drop-offs, and meal preparations, so I could devote uninterrupted hours to research, writing, and editing in my home office.

A very special thank you goes to my boys—Stephen, Camden, and Treyson. They provide me the inspiration to end this pattern of chronic disease for the next generation. I love them so much, and I really want them to grow up in a world where chronic disease is rare, not the norm.

The thing you learn from writing books is that there wouldn't be any on the shelves without the generosity of others. With that, I want to thank Amy Hart, without whom this book would have never crossed the finish line. I had the pleasure of working with Amy on a documentary project where she became a trusted friend and colleague. Amy understood my vision for the book and through her lens as a gifted storyteller she provided invaluable suggestions, edits, and marketing support.

I am forever grateful to Suzanne Darkan, my illustrator, for her willingness to take on the creative elements of a book project from a stranger. Her generosity of time and collaborative spirit brought so much joy to this experience. She went far beyond the creative call of duty. I will always cherish our shared laughs and our new friendship.

I would not be where I am if it weren't for the encouragement of a few people who nurtured me in the beginning stages when things were still very raw. I was working with editor Margot Dougherty on the revised edition of my first book when I decided to move forward with Hay House. Some of Margot's influences are infused in the introduction of this book, and I look forward to working with her again. My editor, Rachel Holtzman, is a saint for returning my e-mails after the reading the first few drafts of my manuscript. Her engaging questions and skillful edits made this book better for sure, but it was her kindness that I will never forget. It really was a mess.

Credit for answering all my random questions and offering generous support goes to literary agents Lindsey Smith at Speilburg Literary Agency and Andrea Barzvi at Empire Literary.

Though it has long been a dream of mine, I never imagined I would actually publish a book with Hay House. I was in discussions with another publisher for another book when I received a call from Hay House, Inc., CEO Reid Tracy. I am grateful for the college professor who told my English literature class that some of the most interesting people in the world major in English and go on to write books. I also owe a great deal to Anne Barthel, the Editorial Director at Hay House, whose guidance kept me going.

I feel very fortunate to be supported by my talented editor Sally Mason-Swaab. Thank you for putting up with me, but most of all, for your diligence and flexibility throughout the process. All of the plans for this book—from the cover design to the copyediting to the final distribution—were assembled by a dedicated team at Hay House including Marlene Robinson, Celeste Johnson, Byron Campbell, and Patricia Gift, for which I am grateful.

Special thanks to my dear friend Bella Lemieux who has a career and a family of her own but who still willingly took the time to read an early draft of my manuscript to keep me moving forward and, as always, cheer me on.

Thank you to all the researchers, practitioners, farmers, advocates, and passionate people who have devoted their careers to regenerating human health and the health of the planet. A special mention goes to Didi Pershouse who indirectly contributed to this work by writing and gifting me a copy of her book, *The Ecology of Care,* which reignited my soul. This was the reminder I didn't know I needed that other professional women in the health field felt the way I did about the intelligence of the whole and our need to heal as a community.

ABOUT THE AUTHOR

As a nutrition educator and researcher, Kathleen has dedicated her work to increasing the public's knowledge about patterns of disease and our innate capacity to heal. Kathleen is a Functional Diagnostic Nutrition Practitioner and Certified Integrative Health & Nutrition Coach with specialized training in biochemistry for autism, allergies, autoimmune, and chronic conditions. She is the Founder of the Nutritional Intelligence Academy and serves as an adviser to many organizations. Kathleen is a well-respected national speaker and has been featured on a wide range of media outlets including international broadcasts. She is the author of *The Hidden Connection* and the main feature in the award-winning documentary film *Secret Ingredients*. She lives in Rhode Island with her husband and three sons.

Learn: www.kathleendichiara.com
Follow: @Kathleendichiara

ABOUT THE ILLUSTRATOR

Suzanne Darkan is a London-based illustrator and founder of Doodles For Change. For more information on Suzanne's work visit www.doodlesforchange.co.uk.

We hope you enjoyed this Hay House book. If you'd like to receive our online catalog featuring additional information on Hay House books and products, or if you'd like to find out more about the Hay Foundation, please contact:

Hay House, Inc., P.O. Box 5100, Carlsbad, CA 92018-5100
(760) 431-7695 or (800) 654-5126
(760) 431-6948 (fax) or (800) 650-5115 (fax)
www.hayhouse.com® • www.hayfoundation.org

———

Published in Australia by: Hay House Australia Pty. Ltd.,
18/36 Ralph St., Alexandria NSW 2015
Phone: 612-9669-4299 • *Fax:* 612-9669-4144
www.hayhouse.com.au

Published in the United Kingdom by: Hay House UK, Ltd.,
The Sixth Floor, Watson House, 54 Baker Street, London W1U 7BU
Phone: +44 (0)20 3927 7290 • *Fax:* +44 (0)20 3927 7291
www.hayhouse.co.uk

Published in India by: Hay House Publishers India,
Muskaan Complex, Plot No. 3, B-2, Vasant Kunj, New Delhi 110 070
Phone: 91-11-4176-1620 • *Fax:* 91-11-4176-1630
www.hayhouse.co.in

———

Access New Knowledge.
Anytime. Anywhere.

Learn and evolve at your own pace
with the world's leading experts.

www.hayhouseU.com

Hay House Titles of Related Interest

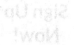